THE NEW MEDICINE

Life and Death after Hippocrates

NEW EDITION

Nigel M. de S. Cameron

FOUNDING EDITOR, *Ethics and Medicine: An International Journal of Bioethics*

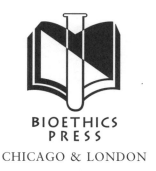

BIOETHICS PRESS

CHICAGO & LONDON

In memory of my mother
and to my father
with love

Contents

'The most fascinating recent comment on the Hippocratic Oath is one which originated with Margaret Mead, the great anthropologist. Her major insight was that the Hippocratic Oath marked one of the turning points in the history of man. She says, "For the first time in our tradition there was a complete separation between killing and curing. Throughout the primitive world the doctor and the sorcerer tended to be the same person. He with the power to kill had power to cure . . . He who had power to cure would necessarily also be able to kill.

' "With the Greeks," says Margaret Mead, "the distinction was made clear. One profession . . . were to be dedicated completely to life under all circumstances, regardless of rank, age, or intellect – the life of a slave, the life of the Emperor, the life of a foreign man, the life of a defective child . . . but society always is attempting to make the physician into a killer – to kill the defective child at birth, to leave the sleeping pills beside the bed of the cancer patient . . . " '

Maurice Levine, *Psychiatry and Ethics*, New York, 1972, quoting a personal communication

The New Medicine
in the Third Millennium

In the decade since this book was issued both medicine and its step-sibling bio-medicine have witnessed extraordinary advance. Yet despite the continued momentum of bioethics, a field whose time has surely come, our Moral uncertainties as a civilization continue to grow at an even faster pace than the nexus of science and medical practice that holds us in such anguished awe. For as new questions are raised, and old given sharper focus and renewed circulation, the capacity of our culture to discover answers that will command a consensus and give us a basis for our common life continues to diminish. The predicament of "the west" as the global leader in both technology and morals is impossible to exaggerate. As our scientific knowledge, especially in the biosciences with their attendant medical-technological capacities, maintains its exponential growth, our moral knowledge, and our capacity therefore to channel and constrain these capacities in the service of humankind, continues to diminish. It is perhaps the supreme and tragic irony of western history that at that moment when the demand for moral vision is at its greatest, its supply is found at its lowest ebb for many hundreds of years.

This view, like some others outlined in *The New Medicine*, is offered in the knowledge that the painter is using a broad brush. The point is to offer perspective, and to do so in a context in which perspective is so often what has been found to be wanting in contemporary discussion. There is a need for fine brushwork also, and some of it is to be found in the pages that follow. Yet what we need above all is a sense of the general direction of things; for our medical-scientific culture is in process of a shift of tectonic proportions. All the many debates and changes in which we are engaged – from the restructuring of "healthcare" delivery and costing, to the human genome project and its fruit – are fundamentally inter-connected.

Only by grasping that fact and its dynamics will we be able to gain perspective on the many particular questions under discussion. The aim of *The New Medicine* when it was first published was to do just that, to offer a powerful framework of understanding within which these many questions could be seen to fall into place. The framework, as the subtitle "Life and Death After Hippocrates" suggests, is that of the Hippocratic medical tradition; to be precise the tradition of "Christian Hippocratism" that has dominated and determined the medical tradition of the western world down nearly two thousand years of history, and that continues, despite very serious challenges, to be an immense influence for good at the turn of the third millennium. By "Christian Hippocratism" we mean, briefly, that amalgam of classical Hippocratic medical values and the Judeo-Christian worldview that has formed the mainstream medical tradition of the western world. It is probably best to use the term "amalgam," since one of the curiosities of the western tradition and, at the same time, a cause of disquiet among Christians today, is the degree to which the pagan origins of Hippocratism were permitted to survive its adoption by Christendom. That in turn has led, among those who have sought in recent years to revive interest in the Hippocratic Oath, to a spate or revisions and re-writes that excise the overtly pagan element. In general, and while we recognize the problem posed by the pagan character of the Oath, this practice is to be discouraged, since it has left us with several fragmented versions of the Oath at a time when fragmentation is at the heart of our problem. (See BioethicsWeb.com for further discussion and various versions of the Oath.)

The argument of the book is, in short, that the incipient collapse of the Hippocratic tradition is leading to the development of a "new medicine" in which the moral vision that has driven medicine is being displaced. Many of the major questions under current discussion are directly related to the Hippocratic collapse, especially those that cluster around the question of the sanctity of life, and that other and seemingly disconnected set that concern the nature of the medical profession and the "delivery" of what is increasingly and most unfortunately termed "healthcare."

The life issues encompass both the old questions of abortion and euthanasia – ancient vices that our ancestors believed the spread of

Judeo-Christian values had put to flight, but that have come back to haunt us as we move beyond the Judeo-Christian moral consensus – and new questions that offer fresh versions of these ancient vices for the brash and pragmatic technological society of the 21st century: options such as deleterious research on the human embryo, and in its latest twist the re-statement of that option in the context of both cloning and research on human stem-cells.

The rapid shifts and uncertain direction in the financing and provision of medical care in many countries, and especially the Unites States, offer a window on one of the most crucial and yet neglected issues in the modern world: the fate of the professions. By a curiously American irony the rise of "managed care" in the United States, quite the most significant feature of which is its concentration of medical provision in the hands of corporations, has delivered Americans from the putative horrors of "socialized medicine" yet by turning medicine into a corporate product. It is a complex and interesting task to weigh the moral and other merits of the varied systems of medical provision. The chief criterion of any such weighing will always be that of "professional alignment" – the degree to which the system upholds or undermines the professional character of the enterprise. By such a criterion, it is hard to avoid the conclusion that the corporatization of medicine is that option least friendly to the professional idea, and arguably more damaging to its flourishing than the more humane and intelligent models of social provision. Thus, when the National Health Service was introduced in the United Kingdom in the aftermath of the Second World War, one of the best decisions taken was to leave family practitioners as self-employed professionals: while the system moved to a single-payer model, its main body of physicians were protected from the worst aspect of such a model in that they did not become civil servants. By the same token, it was the sheer illiberality of the failed Clinton plan of the early 90s that helped secure its doom, with threats (for example) of criminal sanctions for those who sought to deliver and receive medical care outside the ambit of its provision. Let me restate: the central question is that of professional alignment; to what degree is the professional character of medical provision aided or undermined by the systems of financing and management in which it subsists? One reason for posing the question in that manner is to draw attention to the problematic character of traditional western models of medical provision, where the traditional "fee-for-service" approach that was focused on an individual physician in general practice offers an estimable paradigm and yet does so in a context in which the growth of knowledge means that specialization, exponentially increasing costs, and hospital-based practice must also find their place in the medicine of tomorrow.

Needless to say, it is particularly unfortunate that in the many debates of the 1990s about the delivery of medicine, especially in the US and the UK, concern for the professional criterion has been rarely voiced. That is not to say that physicians' "professional" organizations have been silent or inactive. But their concerns have in general related only tangentially to the professional question.

There may seem to be little connection between the corporatization of medicine and key bioethics issues such as the morality of stem-cell and embryo research, but in fact the connection is close. For these questions are being raised in the highly fragmented context of contemporary medicine. Were their location firmly within the professional model, the character of the discussion would be altogether different. But these issues are coming into discussion from one or both of two other directions. At one level, of course, they are posed by developments in the biosciences. While members of the bioscience research community are sometimes physicians as well as researchers, the connection is increasingly accidental. And secondly, they come to their sharpest focus in their corporate context. The biotechnology companies are increasingly setting the pace not simply in their more traditional role of developing the fruit of basic science research, but – more in the manner of pharmaceutical development – now finding themselves at the forefront of basic science. The implications of this development are huge. Among other things, it breaks the near-monopoly of public funding for basic work in the biosciences, and thereby sharpens the issue of the role of public policy. The current US debate over public funding for deleterious research on human stem-cells is a case in point. A prohibition of funding for embryo research had severely curtailed such work in the US. It is now proposed to use stem-cells from privately-funded embryo destruction for publicly-funded research. Or again, take the role of Celera Genomics in rivaling the publicly-funded Human Genome Project as the work of mapping the genome has accelerated toward completion. In this context, professional supervision of the basic science and application development is entirely absent; supervision through public policy becomes increasingly difficult. The corporatization of the biosciences stands in parallel with that of medical provision through the "profession." Medicine is being steadily redefined as a consumer product, and corporate structures put in place to shape, market, and deliver the product to its consumers.

In the decade since *The New Medicine* made its first appearance, everything has changed and yet nothing has changed. The gears of massive cultural shift continue to grind; in every nation that traces its roots to the amalgam of classical and Judeo-Christian civilization that we call "the west," the seemingly inexorable process of transformation into a new cultural pattern continues; the trend toward post-Hippocratic medicine moves, however erratically, forward. At the same time, what we might refer to as the clinical heart of medicine – its classic work of therapeutics and palliation – is giving place in both the public imagination and the informed mind of the culture to a fresh center of focus, as the capacity of technology to delight, to impress, to dazzle, and to scare, is demonstrated afresh every day.

Cloning, for example, was a mere sci-fi debating point in 1990. After unprecedented publicity in 1997, when the cloning of Dolly the sheep was announced from Roslin, Scotland, a major opportunity has opened for bioscience research, commercial development, and ultimately medical practice. The challenge to public policy was fundamental and immediate. Efforts to ban the birth of cloned babies were unsuccessful at the level of federal legislation in the United States, though led to the addition of a special protocol to the European Convention on Biomedicine and Human Rights. Efforts to prevent the use of somatic-cell nuclear transfer technology to facilitate deleterious research on human embryos are meeting with difficulty, especially in light of the new interest in research on human stem cells, for which an embryo, cloned or otherwise, offers a prime source. Most outrageously, in the United Kingdom the government has moved to use the cloning technique to increase the flow of research embryos.

This is not the place to engage that debate, or to anticipate the incipient challenges from the exploitation of the vast library of information that is even now being mined open-cast in human genetics. Yet these matters lie ahead, on the near horizons of the human race. What should be noted is the extraordinary pace of technological change, and the fact that while technology does not change the basic moral questions that confront its potential beneficiaries, it re-shapes them in such a fashion as to render them both more complex and also more threatening. Never have the questions so elegantly raised by Hippocrates in the centuries before Christ been more relevant than in the third millennium AD. Yet, as couples search for their best choice of gametes on the internet while they "plan" their "family" (how perfect the internet will be for the marketing of clones), and as the stem cell debate seems to have moved beyond any serious interest in the age-old weighing of ends and means, we sample the moral culture of tomorrow. A recent article suggested that computing power in the first 30 years of the new millennium might increase by a factor of one million. The exponential character of developments in the biosciences, correlated as they are with both information technology and venture capitalism, offer a startling prospect. And they throw down the gauntlet to public policy at every level, at a time when we have less and less confidence as a community in the possibility of moral consensus as the basis for our common life.

Yet Hippocrates remains the patient's friend, locking every aspect of medical practice into the transcendent web of moral vision that brings the human and the divine into a common embrace; that holds physicians accountable one to another in the guild-profession that is thereby constituted; that sets the sanctity and dignity of human life at center-stage. Only thus has humane medicine flourished, and it is hard to see how in any other way it shall flourish again.

Resources related to *The New Medicine* will be found at BioethicsWeb.com and TheCloningDebate.com, together with links to bioethics centers and other sites.

Nigel M. de S. Cameron
info@BioethicsWeb.com

Foreword

The closing years of the twentieth century are a time in which we have very high expectations for medicine and health. We put a great deal of faith in new technologies, new surgical procedures, and new pharmaceuticals. And we continue to have faith in what I call the 'magic' of medicine. We expect miracles to happen – even when the real world of medicine is not always able to deliver.

The delivery of health care today is not what we intended – nor is it what we like. The United Kingdom is attempting to repair or replace a tired national health service. Canada's citizens – once delighted with their health care – are complaining about long waiting lists before diagnosis or treatment, and are dismayed that some patients die before they can receive help. The United States has a crisis in health care: millions have no access to any at all, others get only rationed care, even though rationing has never been publicly discussed. Health insurance resembles a shell game.

But central to all this is the failure of the doctor–patient relationship. Some say cause, others say effect: both are correct. Ethics enjoys a role in the trades, in business and in the professions which it has never had before.

Medicine, more than all the rest, finds its time-honored, almost automatic decisions being referred to medical ethicists – a new and growing breed of professionals – because the members of society no longer share the same values.

We don't know as much as we would like to about the practice of medicine or what doctors did in, say, 400 BC. But we do know there was then, as now, a broad spectrum of behavior, personal and professional, especially revealed in the way doctors treated patients. Then, as now, there were significant differences in values.

The emergence of the age of Hippocrates saw a band of physicians set themselves apart to lead exemplary lives, indeed, pure and holy lives, in reference to their profession (their teachers *et al*) and to their patients. They asked their pagan gods to be witnesses to their resolve; they believed they deserved to live in dishonor if they forswore their oath and promise. They started as a minority movement in the healing art, but their influence spread; the Hippocratic tradition was born and served us well for several millennia.

In the post-World-War-II era in western civilization, an equally important but opposite trend began to evolve. Physicians began to water down the basic tenets of the Hippocratic tradition, and then they abandoned them. This time there was a band of physicians who remained faithful to the old traditions and watched their numbers diminish. Today, again, they are a minority in the healing art. Their influence is less important than it used to be. How will patients be served in the future? That's what this book is all about: the rise and fall of Hippocratic medicine. Where *should* we go? Where *will* we go?

In Cameron's view the *sine qua non* of Hippocratic medical practice is the concept of doctor as healer. All else is missing the mark. The doctor can't be the healer he should be without the Hippocratic concept of the sanctity of human life. The Hippocratic Oath was a pagan oath, which it remains to this day. Cameron's genius is that he has put it in a Christian context. The Christian perspective and the Hippocratic Oath are seen as parallel in intent. After reading the Appendix, 'Towards a Theology of Medicine', one may wish to see it expanded to become seminal to a new Christian perspective in health.

What is found in these pages has been tested by the author in conferences and previous journal articles, has stood the test of at least some time, and has the advantage of being the author's second and subsequent thoughts on the issues. There are two areas where disagreement with Cameron's excellent analysis may arise: the 'relief of human suffering' and 'letting nature take its course'.

The oath of Hippocrates is silent on human suffering, whereas the relief of human suffering is the substance of medicine today.

That in itself is odd because in the early days of the Hippocratic school cure was unlikely and palliation, or the relief of suffering, was all the ancient physician really had to offer. However, as a Christian physician who practiced in the Hippocratic tradition, I can say it is quite possible in modern medicine to be committed above all to the sanctity of human life, and yet to relieve suffering in the context of that commitment so that the oath is never abrogated.

Letting nature take its course can mean many different things to different people. When, in the course of illness, do you make this decision? Is it before, during, or after everything known to the healer has been tried? The point is that letting nature take its course is semantically equivalent to the resolve not to prolong the patient's act of dying, but sometimes is semantically a synonym for euthanasia. Again, as a Christian physician, letting nature take its course does not have to be at variance with the oath.

The concept of doctor as healer above all else does not exclude the prevention of disease. Some analysts say that prevention and health promotion can postpone up to 70 per cent of all premature deaths, whereas the traditional curative and reparative approach to medicine can postpone no more than 10–15 per cent of such deaths. Even if they are only half-right, that is quite a difference in social pay-offs.

Even though written in the context of the Christian faith, Cameron's work could be the rallying point for that large segment of the medical profession that may not share Cameron's Christian insight, but who know something is wrong. I have taught Hippocratic principles to medical students for years but I'm going to make a change in my teaching habit. I'm going to seek out pre-med students and acquaint them with the departure from the ordinary that the disciples of Hippocrates left to their posterity. The future doctor must hear the precepts four to eight years earlier than he or she does now. It could make a difference.

C. Everett Koop, MD
Formerly Surgeon-General,
Public Health Service, USA

Introduction

Few people can be unaware of the fact that there are profound ethical problems relating to the practice of medicine in modern times, none more so than in the sphere of human reproduction. Ethical issues have become of far greater relevance to the present generation than for many centuries. Until recently, medicine has been practised – in the western world, at any rate – within the framework, covenant or code (whatever term you use), embodied in the Hippocratic tradition.

Hippocratism was of course a pagan concept, born no doubt from a revulsion against many of the utilitarian practices existing even as late as the fourth century BC, in the era known as 'the glory that was Greece'. Plato enumerates many of these practices with approbation – abortion of the unwanted fetus, exposure of the deformed or handicapped neonate so that it might die. In relation to the adult:

> And therefore our politic Asclepius may be supposed to have exhibited his art to persons who by being of a generally healthy constitution and habit of life had a definite ailment; such as these he cures and has them live as usual, herein consulting the interest of the State. But bodies that disease has penetrated through and through he would not have attempted to cure. He did not want to lengthen out good-for-nothing lives or to have weak fathers begetting weaker sons. If a man was not able to live in the ordinary way he had no business to cure him, for such a cure would have been no use either to himself or to the State.

Although pagan in origin, the Hippocratic tradition gradually became strengthened through the Judaeo–Christian belief in the sanctity of human life. The physician, in healing the sick, forbore to do anything to harm his patient, and accepted that he must never administer 'a poison to anyone if asked to do so' – the most common form of suicide–euthanasia in the ancient world.

Today, therefore, by accepting liberal abortion, contemplating experimentation on the human fetus, being ambivalent about the question of allowing the handicapped neonate to die and about euthanasia, is medicine abandoning Hippocratism?

In many respects the answer, obviously, is yes. The medical profession has found it increasingly difficult to maintain its hitherto ethical practice in these areas against the pressures of an increasingly agnostic state, and public attitudes. The medical professions in most countries which have adopted liberal abortion were at first hostile to legislation. However, all but a minority soon abandoned these principles and have presided over the killing of millions of fetuses. All attempts to modify liberal legislation have been vigorously resisted. So much for the Hippocratic injunction not to assist a woman to procure an abortion – and indeed for the ethical code of the World Medical Association which, until recently, required the doctor to have the utmost respect for human life from the time of conception.

Is the fetus human? That is the fundamental issue in the current debate about experimentation on the fetus (embryo). If the fetus can be destroyed so easily for often trivial reasons, to satisfy the wishes of the mother, why worry about using the embryo as an experimental animal? Why not indeed, if you deny the humanness of the fetus and are prepared to introduce veterinary practices into controlled and assisted human reproduction.

But it is paradoxical, indeed ironic, that at the very time when medical scientists are anxious to use the embryo for experiments designed not to benefit that embryo but others, we also have an expanding discipline referred to as 'fetal medicine'. Modern technology is making it possible not only to investigate the well-being of the fetus *in utero*, but also to treat it. Neo-natal intensive care is saving many lives that would have been lost previously. Surely this must implicitly acknowledge the humanness of the fetus. How shall we decide which fetus shall be experimented upon, which killed and which saved? The present policy of 'diagnose and destroy' the abnormal or handicapped fetus is only one step removed from neo-natal killing and ignores fundamental moral issues.

Dr Cameron in this book on the 'new medicine' has produced a most valuable contribution to the debate about ethical and moral issues in modern medicine. He writes as a theologian, but he has a remarkable knowledge of the details of medical practices not always evident in others who comment on these subjects. His text is beautifully written and very extensively researched. He writes with frankness and candour and spells out in detail the ethical problems involved in the medical practices to which he refers.

In saying that 'the leadership of the profession is now in the hands of a generation which knew not Hippocrates,' he is perhaps too harsh – but it needs saying, even though it does not apply to all. He acknowledges that those who criticise the new medicine are in the position of a beleaguered minority, and that it may appear to be a tall order to take on our contemporary post-Hippocratic society. But he believes that because the western world owes an enormous debt to the Christian tradition, it is right to challenge the post-Christian ideas of the western world. His goal is the recovery of a Hippocratic medical culture, which contains the extraordinary advances in medical techniques which have brought so many benefits, within Hippocratic medical values. It is a goal worth striving for, and I welcome Dr Cameron's scholarly contribution to a debate that is far from over.

Sir John Peel, KCVO
Past President, British Medical Association

1

The Hippocratic Legacy

Medicine is so closely linked with the name of Hippocrates that it seems hard to believe that they could ever be put asunder. Even today – despite everything in the following chapters – our medical tradition still clings to his name, so that every statement of medical values either consciously or unconsciously follows the form of the Hippocratic Oath. Yet the argument of this book is that after Hippocrates – when medicine departs from the values of the Oath and ceases to be Hippocratic – it loses something essential to its character; in fact, it begins to cease to be 'medicine' at all.

This claim rests on a particular understanding of what, in essence, medicine *is*. Plainly, a doctor may reject every principle of the Hippocratic tradition and still remain skilled in clinical practice. Is it not this clinical expertise that constitutes medicine, and the exercise of skill that makes a doctor a doctor?

The real question is this: is medicine essentially a matter of medical technique? Or is it, rather, a matter of values, of moral commitments in the exercise of clinical skills? This issue is explored in some detail in the next chapter. First we set the scene by enquiring into the character of the 'medicine' that we have inherited in the Hippocratic tradition. Although Hippocrates remains one of the best-known names from the ancient world, many doctors have only a hazy notion of what he has meant for their profession. Modern scholarly discussion has cast fresh light on the origins and character of the blend of clinical practice and ethics which we associate with his name and which marks the starting-point of our medical tradition. However, Hippocrates himself remains obscure, and we now know that many, if not all, of the writings attributed to him were the work of later disciples. Yet while we know little of him, the influence of this colossus of ancient medicine is profound. Not only did he found a loyal 'school' of doctors (perhaps an actual institution, perhaps not), but he also set out to change the basic character of ancient medicine. The ethical pattern of professional practice outlined in the Oath was deeply at odds with the medicine of his time, and it takes on a new relevance today when, once more, it is out of step with mainstream medicine. So what are these values that have so profoundly influenced the direction of western medicine?

THE OATH

We begin with the Hippocratic Oath itself. Although there has been uncertainty about its origins and disagreement over its application, there is little room for controversy about what it actually says.

The Oath reads as follows:

The Covenant

I swear by Apollo Physician, by Asclepius, by Hygeia, by Panaceia, and by all the gods and goddesses, making them witnesses, that I will carry out, according to my ability and judgment, this oath and this indenture:

Duties to Teacher

To regard my teacher in this art as equal to my parents; to make him partner in my livelihood, and when he is in need of money to share mine with him; to consider his offspring equal to my brothers; to teach them this art, if they require to learn it, without fee or indenture; and to impart precept, oral instruction, and all the other learning, to my sons, to the sons of my teacher, and to pupils who have signed the indenture and sworn obedience to the physicians' Law, but to none other.

Duties to Patients

I will use treatment to help the sick according to my ability and judgment, but I will never use it to injure or wrong them.

I will not give poison to anyone though asked to do so, nor will I suggest such a plan. Similarly I will not give a pessary to a woman to cause abortion. But in purity and in holiness I will guard my life and my art.

I will not use the knife either on sufferers from stone, but will give place to such as are craftsmen therein.

Into whatsoever house I enter, I will do so to help the sick, keeping myself free from all intentional wrong-doing and harm, especially from fornication with woman or man, bond or free.

Whatsoever in the course of practice I see or hear (or even outside my practice in social intercourse) that ought never to be published abroad, I will not divulge, but consider such things to be holy secrets.

The Sanction

Now if I keep this oath and break it not, may I enjoy honour, in my life and art, among all men for all time; but if I transgress and forswear myself, may the opposite befall me.[1]

As we see, the Oath breaks naturally into three main sections (the opening invocation of the gods and the sanction at the end should be taken together). The central, ethical sections deal respectively with the physician's duties to his teacher and to his patients. This latter part is the most familiar today; the others read rather strangely and, in the many modern statements of medical values in which the Oath is taken as a model, they have been excised or substantially altered. Yet despite the primacy of the more obviously professional obligations, it would be a mistake to regard the rest as irrelevant. The Hippocratic Oath comes down to us as a package. And since its role in forming and developing the western medical tradition has been so immense, it demands consideration in all its parts. In fact those clauses of questionable relevance are far from unimportant. Each one has played its own strategic part in determining the direction of the medical tradition.

The Doctor and his Patients

The doctor's promises relating to his treatment of his patients have always been seen as the central elements in the Oath. Here we find the doctor's role and calling defined; the negatively phrased series of 'I will not' clauses actually mark out positively the area in which the physician is to fulfil his calling. It defines the character of the healing task.

I will use treatment to help the sick according to my ability and judgment, writes Hippocrates, *but I will never use it to injure or wrong them.* To our modern minds, this first solemn declaration in relation to patient care seems so plainly acceptable as to be almost trivial. We have become very used to the idea that a doctor should use his skills and opportunities in the interest of healing his patient. But our familiarity has been bred precisely by the influence of the Hippocratic tradition. Hippocratic medicine 'goes without saying' because we still look out across the landscape of a Hippocratic world.

Perhaps the best illustration of the Hippocratic character of our perceptions is to be found in an important book on the Oath published in the 1920s. According to W. H. S. Jones in *The Doctor's Oath*: 'Custom and convenience, to say nothing of the human conscience, would sooner or later lay down most of the rules of conduct comprised in *Oath*' (with the lone exception of the clause on operations for bladder stones).[2]

If Jones were writing today it would be difficult for him to speak in this curiously complacent way. Familiarity has long bred a respect for Hippocrates which has become largely a matter of form. Medical students, for example, have no more than a nodding acquaintance with the Oath and the questions it raises; and scholarly discussion – in a field which has long had a keen interest in its own history and development – has been limited.

In fact, like so much else in the Oath which Jones found commonplace, the physician's commitment to his patient is a distinguishing mark of this particular medical tradition. Hippocratic medicine is characterised by the physician's setting his 'ability and judgment' at the sole disposal of the interests of his patient. Lest there be any misunderstanding, the point is made first positively, then negatively: 'I will never use it [treatment] to injure or wrong' the sick. Then the two specific clinical implications of this clause are spelled out, first in respect of euthanasia.

I will not give poison to anyone though asked to do so, nor will I suggest such a plan. The taking of poison was the commonest means of suicide in ancient Greece, and the physician (who apparently often acted as his own pharmacist) was asked to assist. In a primitive medical context, without the aid of the panoply of modern developments in surgery and drug therapy, the resort to suicide was not uncommon and filled the role of voluntary euthanasia today. It was a society in which suicide itself was widely approved. In this first substantive ethical commitment, the Hippocratic physician repudiates such an approach to sickness and death. Even though asked to do so, he will not prescribe poison nor ever suggest such a resolution of the dreadful dilemma of chronic and terminal disease.

In spelling out one implication of the physician's refusal – even 'though asked to do so' – to injure his patient, the Oath makes plain his commitment to the idea that the doctor knows best. His system of values must be accepted by the patient. Here is a plain case in which the patient asks for a specific form of help, and the doctor says no. The fact that this practice was not then illegal, indeed was widely approved, offers plain evidence of the distinctive character of the specific ethical tradition to which the Hippocratic physician was committed. This becomes even clearer when we turn to the following clause.

Similarly I will not give a pessary to a woman to cause abortion.

Many of those who debate abortion today, pro and con, are ignorant of the ancient character of the argument – and the practice. Abortion was common in the permissive society of the Graeco-Roman world, and, as we see here, the most common means of inducing it was by the insertion of a pessary (just as the most common means of suicide was poison). Like suicide–euthanasia, it was something which specially concerned the physician, since physicians' abortion services were in demand (for the same wide range of reasons for which they are sought today).

It is interesting to note that in one later revision of the Oath (a 'Christian version') the abortion clause is extended to cover abortion 'from above or from below',[3] turning it into a comprehensive proscription of all contemporary abortion methods (pessaries, oral abortifacients, surgery), perhaps owing to the increasing popularity of methods other than the pessary and attempts by physicians to get around the Oath's prohibitions. It is plain, however, that (like the reference to poison in the preceding clause) the one method is intended to stand for them all. Hippocratic medicine was inimical to abortion, as it was to any suicide or euthanasia, however caused or for whatever reason.

That section of the Oath concludes in these terms of contrast: *But in purity and in holiness I will guard my life and my art.* We will return later to the religious character of the Oath, but it is evident, even at this stage, that its religious context is not confined to the formal elements of the opening and closing sections. Hippocratic ethics, as we might say, is theistic – even theological – ethics. Its character depends on theological premises. The physician's rejection of any use of his skills 'to injure or wrong' his patients (specifically, to assist in or suggest suicide–euthanasia, or to procure abortion) is all part of living a pure and holy life. For him to pull back from the emphatic Hippocratic rejection of these misuses of his skills would be to render him 'impure' and 'unholy' – in his 'life' as in his 'art'. Two enlightening conclusions then follow.

Firstly, we note that some kind of ethical 'paternalism' is fundamental to the Hippocratic concept of medicine. The Hippocratic physician engages to practise a specific kind of medicine; not whatever kind of medicine the marketplace demands. His interest is not primarily in how his patient sees things; and he finds it impossible to believe that his patient's true interests could actually lie in any other direction than that to which by oath he is committed. The society in which the Hippocratic Oath was first sworn was profoundly pluralistic, and that was the context in which the Oath invited the physician to commit himself to one particular set of values. His answer to pluralism did not lie in relativising his own moral and professional commitments and seeking to adapt them to those of his patients. Indeed, the whole purpose of the Oath was to meet the challenge of a plurality of religious and ethical convictions by calling on the physician to assert and practise one particular option among the many. We return to this question in Chapter Six.

Secondly, we note that the Hippocratic physician is a professional (though in almost the reverse of the sense in which the term is often used today, where it means 'detached'; 'merely professional'). This is a fundamental element in the Hippocratic pattern, the synthesis of 'life' and 'art'. Once a physician, always a physician; a physician through and through. The taking of the Oath is akin to an act of ordination, the setting apart of this one individual for a special purpose. In this respect, as in others, Hippocratic medicine blazes the trail which the other professions have followed in their own fashion. Indeed, it could be argued that medicine is the profession *par excellence*, and other professions are professions only by extension or analogy. The physician's dedicated life intermingles with his skilful practice of the medical arts. By oath, the 'purity and holiness' of the physician's life and of his art are linked in indissoluble marriage.

And these two conclusions are intimately connected, for the self-involving moral logic of Hippocratic medicine demands a set of moral commitments which are not negotiable. The physician is set apart to practise medicine according to highly distinctive canons. He is thereby committed not merely in general terms, to refrain from injury or wrong to his patients, but to refrain from injury or wrong as set out and defined in the Oath. The purpose, of course, is to offer a sufficiently careful ethical definition of medicine to ensure its distinctive continuance in a context of pluralism, in which there is fundamental disagreement about right and wrong in medicine, as in every other aspect of social life. In such a context, not only is the medical tradition under pressure, but so is the individual doctor. It is partly for these reasons that the Oath is of such relevance today.

There then follows the clause which has most puzzled interpreters of the oath: *I will not use the knife either [or even] on sufferers from stone, but will give place to such as are craftsmen therein.* The contrast between this statement and the preceding statements about abortion and suicide–euthanasia is striking. Whatever the reason that lies behind Hippocrates' repudiation of surgery (specifically, for bladder stones though, as with poison and pessaries, its treatment presumably stands for all surgery), the objection cannot be, as in those cases, on grounds of principle, for provision is made for 'referral' to a surgeon. So this cannot be an objection to surgery as such, but simply to its practice by the physician. This clause is thought to have been influential in separating surgery and internal medicine in medical history, though the reasoning behind it is far from clear. Perhaps the best explanation lies in reading it as a commendation of specialisation and referral in the interests of competence. The physician should not dabble (greedily?) in this special skill but concentrate on medicine proper.

Into whatsoever house I enter, I will do so to help the sick, keeping myself free from all intentional wrong-doing and harm, especially from fornication with woman or man, bond or free.

In this clause and the next the Oath continues with its theme of 'in purity and in holiness' – the union of medical skill and integrity of person – as the keystone of the Hippocratic vocation. The privilege and intimacy of access which are necessarily given the physician in the conduct of his professional life offer him two kinds of privileged opportunity to abuse his professional relationships. The first is under scrutiny here: that of engaging in 'intentional wrong-doing and harm' in the home of his patient. Sexual opportunity is singled out as an obvious route to abuse and is duly blocked, although, as the Oath implies, this is simply one striking example of the physician's opportunity for misconduct. It is interesting to note the Oath's blanket proscription of sexual relations in 'whatsoever houses' the physician enters. The ban does not cover the patient only, but all those in the household, since the reason why the physician has access to them lies in his vocation. Moreover, it extends even to the slaves of the household. Whatever may be his own private sexual *mores* (and the implication of this clause is that they will not necessarily involve abstinence from 'fornication'), his professional life must be carefully circumscribed.

The second area of opportunity which the physician forswears is found in the following clause: *Whatsoever in the course of practice I see or hear (or even outside my practice in social intercourse) that ought never to be published abroad, I will not divulge, but consider such things to be holy secrets.* His privilege of access leads him to refuse opportunities for 'intentional wrong-doing';

and it leads him also to treat what he 'sees and hears' in the course of his professional practice as privileged information. There are several aspects to this clause. For one thing, the commitment to confidentiality is not limited to a refusal to abuse information, in line with the previous clause's refusal to abuse relationships and opportunities for wrong-doing. It clearly goes beyond that into a broad, and remarkably contemporary, concept of privacy. Indeed, it is even broader than we might expect, since it specifically includes information gained by the physician in his private life, outside the context of professional access.

That the Oath should spell this out underlines the remarkably high standards which the physician is expected to maintain, and offers a further reminder of the unity of life and art in the Hippocratic vocation. The ban covers not only what is revealed to the doctor in the course of the professional consultation, but anything which may come to his notice which could affect the interests of his patient. The doctor–patient relationship implicit in the Oath involves the wholesale commitment of the physician to his patient's interests. The professional relationship extends, as it were, round the clock. The physician is never able to look at his patient as if he were anything other than his patient. Just as he is 'once a physician, always a physician', so a patient, once a patient, has never anything other than a privileged relationship with him.

Yet this is no absolute ban. The Oath refers to information 'which ought not to be published abroad'. This could allow for knowledge professionally disclosed (for example, in referral), but could also cover circumstances in which either the patient's own interests or his obligations to others suggested that confidentiality should deliberately be breached (if, perhaps, he is epileptic, or schizophrenic – or HIV positive, and cannot be persuaded to tell those who ought to know). We may be tempted to read too much into the Oath, but in so carefully crafted a document this phrase may well bear such a meaning.

Yet, as a general principle, information about his patient is not simply secret, it is a 'holy secret'; to divulge or exploit such information, the Oath here reminds the physician, is to commit a crime against the God in whose name the Oath is sworn. His patient's secrets are *God's* secrets. This is a truly remarkable doctrine of medical confidentiality!

The Doctor and his Teacher

The Oath must first have been intended to be used in a school or guild in which its ethical principles were passed on from teacher to pupil, along with the body of clinical expertise. This is the situation to which the clauses of the Oath dealing with pupil–teacher relations chiefly refer. We read of the profound respect which underlies this relationship, and the deep seriousness with which the newcomer views his indenture. And we learn more of the 'professional' character of the medical enterprise.

To regard my teacher in this art as equal to my parents; to make him partner in my livelihood, and when he is in need of money to share mine with him; to consider his offspring equal to my brothers; to teach them this art, if they require to learn it, without fee or indenture; and to impart precept, oral instruction, and all the other learning, to my sons, to the sons of my teacher, and to pupils who have signed the indenture and sworn obedience to the physicians' Law, but to none other.

This section provides for the continuation of the Hippocratic school, and regulates relations between teacher and pupil. The pupil is in some way taken into the household of his teacher, such that his relations with the teacher and with the teacher's children are the equivalent of a son's with his parents and siblings. He takes on an obligation to work in partnership with his teacher, if need be to support him, and to teach his children free of charge. And he is obliged also to pass on the Hippocratic tradition to his own sons and to indentured pupils (who presumably pay a fee). Yet such indentured pupils must have 'sworn obedience to the physicians' Law' (another name for the Oath). The Oath explicitly forbids the physician to pass on his clinical knowledge to anyone who has not already committed himself to the Hippocratic values. It is clear from this statement that, contrary to general belief, the Oath was meant to be sworn prior to indenture. This contrasts with modern use of the Oath and re-formulated statements of medical ethics at the end of the process of medical education. Here the requirement is for moral commitment to the Hippocratic code at its outset, a requirement that no doubt reflects the pluralism of ancient Greek society. Nothing may be taken for granted of the aspiring physician.

As we seek to unfold the logic of Hippocratism, we must underline the last four words of this section, 'but to none other'. Like so much else in the Oath, they address the situation of ethical conflict which was characteristic of the religious and philosophical diversity of the Greece of late antiquity as it is of ours today. By these four words the Oath strictly commits the physician (and the medical student) to secrecy concerning the entire body of clinical medicine. It is to be made available only to those who have first committed themselves to the Hippocratic ethical framework. From the point of view of those who first framed and swore the Oath, medical practice and stringent Hippocratic values had always to go together.

The Doctor and his God(s)

We turn now to the third strand in the Oath, the 'oath proper' which sandwiches the ethical injunctions together. It is in two parts: the invocation of the gods at the beginning, and the sanction of the Oath at the end. Such a pattern was common in the ancient world, and we know that oaths of this kind were particularly common in Greece.

> *I swear by Apollo Physician, by Asclepius, by Hygeia, by Panaceia, and by all the gods and goddesses, making them witnesses, that I will carry out, according to my ability and judgment, this oath and this indenture . . .*
> *Now if I keep this oath and break it not, may I enjoy honour, in my life and art, among all men for all time; but if I transgress and forswear myself, may the opposite befall me.*

The opening words of the Oath remind us forcibly that this document has come down to us from ancient, pagan Greece. Widespread use of the Oath down the Christian centuries must not obscure its original context in pre-Christian pagan antiquity. Yet this well illustrates the universality of the Oath's prescription for medicine. Whatever the details of its religious–philosophical origins (we discuss them below), its overtly pagan milieu has not limited its application in Christian (and other religious) contexts. The calling as witnesses of the deities of Greek paganism has been left to serve a formal function (although, as we see below, in Islam the Oath was revised to disinfect it of such pagan associations). The Oath-form of the document points up the fundamental character of the ethical commitments demanded of the physician. In Greek religion the most solemn sanction lay in summoning the appropriate gods – Apollo, Asclepius, Hygeia, Panaceia.

In this way, the two horizontal relationships in the life of the physician, with his teacher and with his patients, are set in the context of his vertical relationship, with his gods. He is held accountable to them for his relations with teacher and patients. He must answer to them, and he seeks their approval and reward. The ethical monotheism of the Judaeo–Christian tradition could readily absorb such a pattern of theological–ethical understanding, though by infusing it with new meaning which made special sense of the extraordinary Hippocratic values. In the context of the pagan religion of the Oath, medical ethics rise from the flimsiest of pagan theological structures, yet these structures are adequate for their purpose of setting the medical values in a theistic context. I am accountable to the gods for my treatment of my patient, the physician is able to say; the patient's secrets are holy secrets; and so on. Jew and Christian (and Muslim too) could later add their own reasoning: in every patient I find one who bears the image of God himself. The vertical dimension of the physician's ethics is present already in pagan Hippocratism, with its key concept of a responsibility that reaches beyond the doctor–patient relationship to the relationship of both doctor and patient with the gods in whom they believe and who will hold them to account. We return to this question later.

HIPPOCRATES AND HIS SCHOOL

But who was Hippocrates? The *New Oxford Illustrated Dictionary* answers memorably: 'the most famous of all physicians, of whom almost nothing is known.'[4] Who wrote the Hippocratic Oath? Traditionally, of course, the answer was simply 'Hippocrates of Cos', but in recent years a new approach to the question has been developed. It proves to be of considerable value to us in our understanding of the Oath. Indeed, as we shall argue, it sets the question of the role and importance of the Oath today in a fresh perspective of particular contemporary relevance.

The Hippocrates of History

Though the earliest manuscripts of the Oath date from the late Middle Ages, we know of Hippocrates and his physicians from earlier sources. The first indisputable reference is in the works of Scribonius Largus, from the first half of the first century AD. He calls Hippocrates 'the founder of our profession'.[5] But centuries earlier we read of a Hippocrates in one of the plays of Aristophanes. Euripides is asked by Mnesilochus to swear to help him. Euripides agrees: 'I swear then by aether, abode of Zeus.' Mnesilochus retorts: 'Why, rather than by the community of Hippocrates?' Some commentators suggest that another Hippocrates is intended, but Jones, the translator of the Loeb edition of the Hippocratic corpus, concludes that 'it is likely' that Aristophanes was referring to Hippocrates the physician (and the collection of gods referred to at the start of the Oath). That would take the Oath back firmly to at least 400 BC.[6] Making a separate, though perhaps less contentious, point Jones adds: 'It is indeed hard to believe that the nucleus, at least, of *Oath* does not go back to the "great" Hippocrates himself.'[7]

Yet the evidence is slender, however attractive the 'legend' of Hippocrates.[8] There are doubts even as to his dates of birth and death, though 460–377 BC are often given. He certainly lived to a great age, and could have died a centenarian (one source claims at 109!). Though we possess biographies, they are far from contemporary and are regarded as unreliable. The tradition associates him with the medical school on the island of Cos, and tells that his father Heraclitus was a physician himself – allegedly a direct descendant of Aesculapius. The assumption has been that this man Hippocrates penned the Oath and formed a school around his distinctive set of medical–ethical principles, which were then widely accepted within the Greek medical community, before being diffused with the spread of Greek medicine around the Graeco–Roman world.

The true story may be less tidy, though nothing in our discussion of the nature of medicine and the significance of the Hippocratic Oath turns on this historical question. Neither is there anything at stake in the discussion of the authenticity of the many books of the so-called 'Hippocratic corpus', the collection of ancient books associated with the name of the physician, which are now widely held to be the work of a number of authors – however much they reflect the genius, no less clinical than ethical, of Hippocrates of Cos.

Who Were the Hippocratic Physicians?

In 1943 a monograph was published as a supplement to the *Bulletin of the History of Medicine* which has fundamentally altered the way in which we understand the origins of Hippocratic medicine. This ground-breaking discussion has been vitally important in establishing and illustrating key facets of early Hippocratic medicine. We shall look at it carefully.

In *The Hippocratic Oath* Ludwig Edelstein confronted head-on the problem of the identity of Hippocrates and the early Hippocratic physicians:

> Uncertainty still prevails concerning the time when the Oath was composed and concerning the purpose for which it was intended. The dates proposed in modern debate vary from the 6th century BC to the 1st century AD. As for the original intent of the manifesto, it is maintained that the Oath was administered in family guilds of physicians; or that it formed the statute of societies of artisans which perhaps were organized in secret; or that it was an ideal program designed without regard for any particular time or place.[9]

Not content with these uncertainties, Edelstein argued from internal evidence – the nature of its teaching – that the Oath may be clearly identified as originating in one of the schools of ancient Greek philosophy, that of the so-called Pythagoreans.

His case is indirect but persuasive. He searches the literature for information on Greek attitudes toward the issues raised in the Oath, and concludes that there is a remarkable resemblance between Hippocratic values and those of the Pythagoreans. His point of departure is the unambiguous position of the Oath on abortion and the provision of poison for suicide–euthanasia. These contrast with vague and general statements about justice, purity and holiness. Here we find definite positions on controversial ethical issues. 'Their interpretation should therefore provide a clue for a historical identification of the views embodied in the Oath of Hippocrates.'[10]

First, Edelstein confirms the concrete context in Greek antiquity of these two practices which the Oath outlaws. 'Under ancient conditions the physician was often presented with the problem of whether or not he should give an abortive remedy.'[11] 'Abortion was practised in Greek times no less than in the Roman era, and it was resorted to without scruple. Small wonder! In a world in which it was held justifiable to expose children immediately after birth, it would hardly seem objectionable to destroy the embryo.'[12]

But what of suicide–euthanasia, as a problem for the medical practitioner? 'Could the doctor ever advise such an act to his patient? In antiquity this was indeed the case. If the sick felt that their pains had become intolerable, if no help could be expected, they often put an end to their own lives. This fact is repeatedly attested and not only in general terms; even the diseases are specified which in the opinion of the ancients gave justification for a voluntary death.'[13] Edelstein continues: 'Moreover, the taking of poison was the most usual means of committing suicide, and the patient was most likely to demand the poison from his physician who was in possession of deadly drugs and knew those which brought about an easy and painless end.'[14]

Edelstein acknowledges that, even if they were incurably ill, the ancient Greeks faced illness in different ways. With bravery or simple resignation, many carried on living despite their suffering. 'Yet the fact remains that throughout antiquity many people preferred voluntary death to endless agony. This form of "euthanasia" was an everyday reality.' So 'it is quite understandable that the Oath deals with the attitude which the physician should take in regard to the possible suicide of his patient. From a practical point of view it was no less important to tell the ancient doctor what to do when faced with such a situation than it was to advise him about cases of abortion.'[15]

But *why?* 'Apparently,' writes Edelstein, 'these prohibitions did not echo the general feeling of the public.'[16] No more were they recognised in law, which was 'indifferent to foeticide' and in some city states actually institutionalised 'self-murder as a relief from illness'.[17]

What is more, the Hippocratic prohibitions do not even echo the general opinions of the medical profession of the day, since 'in antiquity many physicians actually gave their patients the poison for which they asked. Apparently, *qua* physicians, they felt no compunction about doing so . . . As for abortions, many physicians prescribed and gave abortive remedies.'[18]

Edelstein can conclude from his survey of ancient medical practice: 'In short, the strict attitude upheld by the Oath was not uncontested even from the medical point of view. In antiquity it was not generally considered a violation of medical ethics to do what the Oath forbade. An ancient doctor who accepted the rules laid down by "Hippocrates" was by no means in agreement with the opinion of all his fellow physicians . . . '[19]

Given the mythology which has surrounded the historical questions raised by the Oath and the other writings of the Hippocratic corpus, this clear conclusion is extremely valuable. It has not been seriously contested, and offers a new way of understanding the Hippocratic tradition. From the start, the Hippocratics were a minority, a reforming movement whose distinct professional and ethical characteristics came ultimately to dominate the development of the western medical tradition.

Edelstein associates this movement with the Pythagoreans of the fourth century BC. Here alone does he find a contemporary philosophical school which stood foursquare against suicide. For the Pythagorean, 'suicide was a sin against god who had allocated to man his position in life as a post to be held and to be defended.' So 'in this moral and religious conviction the doctor can well find the courage to remain deaf to his patient's insistence, to his sufferings, and even to the clamour of the world which disagrees almost unanimously with the stand taken by him.'[20]

The same goes for abortion. 'Most of the Greek philosophers even commended abortion.' Yet 'it was different with
the Pythagoreans. They held that the embryo was an animate
being from the moment of conception . . . Consequently, for the
Pythagoreans, abortion, whenever practiced, meant destruction
of a living being.'[21]

Having established these conclusions on the basis of the clauses
of the Oath forbidding abortion and suicide–euthanasia, Edelstein
goes on to argue that the historical context of the remainder of the
Oath lies in the Pythagoreanism of the second half of the fourth
century BC. The striking conclusion which emerges from his
discussion is that Hippocratism does not represent the general
ethical approach to medicine in Greek antiquity. It was controversial from the first. Indeed, 'far from being the expression of
the common Greek attitude towards medicine or of the natural
duties of the physician, the ethical code rather reflects opinions
which were peculiarly those of a small and isolated group.'[22]

And when? Edelstein opts for a date in the later fourth century,
which would place the Oath after the death of Hippocrates. There
must be room for speculation about the relation of the present
form of the Oath and the great physician whose name it bears.
There has long been doubt in respect of the massive corpus of
other literature which has aggregated around his name, some
earlier, some later, but some evidently from this period. For
Edelstein, the later fourth century is in every way a suitable
occasion for the issuing of this reforming medical 'manifesto'.
'In that period many individual attempts were made to improve
medical conditions. Abuses, to be sure, had been criticized even
before. But it is in those Hippocratic treatises that were written
in the second half of the 4th century or even later, that one finds
the first outlines of a system of medical deontology.'[23]

And yet, as time passed, Hippocratism ceased to be the preserve
of only a small minority. In Edelstein's words:

At the end of antiquity a decided change took place. Medical
practice began to conform to that state of affairs which the
Oath had envisaged . . . Now the Oath began to be popular. It
circulated in various forms adapted to the varying circumstances
and purposes of the centuries. Generally considered to be the

work of the great Hippocrates, its study became part of the
medical curriculum . . .

Small wonder! A new religion arose that changed the very
foundations of ancient civilization. Yet, Pythagoreanism seemed
to bridge the gap between heathendom and the new belief.
Christianity found itself in agreement with the principles of
Pythagorean ethics, its concepts of holiness and purity, justice
and forbearance . . . Even the Church Fathers abounded in praise
of the high-mindedness of Hippocrates and his regulations for the
practice of medicine.[24]

Yet, having said all that, Edelstein concludes his study with
these words: 'I venture to suggest that he who undertakes to
study this development [of medical ethics] will find it better
understandable if he realizes that the Hippocratic Oath is a
Pythagorean manifesto and not the expression of an absolute
standard of medical conduct.'[25]

This is a curious contrast, offered as a corrective to the legend
of Hippocrates and the haunting role which his Oath has come
to play in the development of western medicine. By setting
the Pythagorean manifesto over against 'an absolute standard of
moral conduct' at the conclusion of a lengthy scholarly argument,
Edelstein takes the reader by surprise. We comment later on the
role which Edelstein's treatise was called upon to play in the
landmark *Roe v. Wade* judgment of the United States Supreme
Court, who used the Pythagorean identification to justify just
such a relativising of Hippocratic values. Yet to set its prov-
enance in fourth century Pythagoreanism against the notion that
it represents 'the expression of an absolute standard of medical
conduct' is to tilt at a windmill. If Hippocratism had achieved
in fourth century Greece the representative status it did actually
come to bear in later times, it would have shown itself no less,
but no more, deserving of respect; the respect of those who, in
the twentieth century, trace their medical tradition all the way
back to what Edelstein himself has christened 'the first outlines
of a system of medical deontology'.[26]

Indeed, is this distinctive tradition not the *more* worthy of
respect when it is considered that it arose as the manifesto of a
small, reforming minority, who went on to capture the consensus
of the medical tradition of a later generation? Edelstein is less than

candid to imply that it was simply the rise of Christianity, the 'new religion', which through its congruence with Pythagorean ethics turned a sectarian medical creed into the basis of the medical tradition of a civilisation. As Edelstein has himself argued elsewhere, the genius of Hippocratism had secured wide acceptance for its principles among the varieties of Greek paganism long before the conversion of Constantine heralded the triumph of Christianity – and, with it, the baptism of pagan Hippocratism as a Christian medical creed.

Whether or not the Hippocratic Oath represents an 'absolute standard of medical conduct' is another matter. No doubt it did to the Pythagoreans. For many of their successors also, the Oath represents a divine prescription for the human vocation of the physician. Yet the rise and near-universal spread of what Edelstein characterises as a sectarian manifesto owes its influence chiefly to the mesmeric moral power of its ethic.

CHRISTIAN AND MUSLIM ADAPTATIONS

An Early Christian Version

We know that the Oath circulated in a specially Christianised version (or versions) early in the history of the Church. One such version first saw publication in Jones' book *The Doctor's Oath*, although its significance remains uncertain. Jones was in a good position to assess the manuscript evidence for the text of the Oath, and it was his judgment that in antiquity it had various forms mostly lost to us, since the main type of the text reflected in our manuscripts eventually predominated and drove out the others.

The fact that Christian versions were composed and, presumably, used, is a striking indication of the congruence of the ethical kernel of the Oath with the Christian faith. It is interesting to note that we find this version of the Oath written in the manuscript in the shape of a cross.

This is Jones' translation:[27]

> *From the Oath according to Hippocrates in so far as a Christian may swear it.*

Blessed be God the Father of our Lord Jesus Christ, who is blessed for ever and ever; I lie not.

I will bring no stain upon the learning of the medical art. Neither will I give poison to anybody though asked to do so, nor will I suggest such a plan. Similarly I will not give treatment to women to cause abortion, treatment neither from above nor from below. But I will teach this art, to those who require to learn it, without grudging and without an indenture. I will use treatment to help the sick according to my ability and judgment. And in purity and in holiness I will guard my art. Into whatsoever houses I enter, I will do so to help the sick, keeping myself free from all wrong-doing, intentional and unintentional, tending to death or to injury, and from fornication with bond or free, man or woman. Whatsoever in the course of practice I see or hear (or outside my practice in social intercourse) that ought not to be published abroad, I will not divulge, but consider such things to be holy secrets. Now if I keep this oath and break it not, may God be my helper in my life and art, and may I be honoured among men for all time. If I keep faith, well; but if I forswear myself may the opposite befall me.

This revision represents a rather unhappy marriage of the familiar text of the Oath and recognisably Christian sentiments. It does not actually re-state the medical ethics of the Oath in Christian terms. To take a small example, the 'may I be honoured among men for all time' of the penultimate sentence, culled from the original, reads strangely in a Christian document – however plain (indeed, symbolic) is its significance in the pagan original. This no doubt indicates the veneration with which the Hippocratic tradition was already regarded by Christians at the time when this revision was drafted. Here was no attempt to displace Hippocratism with a Christian alternative, but rather to graft the nascent Christian medical tradition on to ancient pagan stock. More important, the covenantal relationship between teacher and pupil which forms part of the structure of the original (and derives from its use as an oath of initiation) is almost entirely lost.

Yet the baptising of the Oath into a 'Christian' document – to which these manuscripts bear witness – underlines Christian respect for its moral force. It is striking that no attempt is made to 'improve' on the medical values of the Oath – to make it more

Christian, as it were. Its ethical structure remains intact, and the only addition is found in the expansion of the abortion clause, to cover other methods than that of the pessary. This no doubt represents the closing of a loophole in the light of contemporary practice (rather than a specifically Christian amendment). It may possibly represent a variant in the text of the pagan Oath itself.

There are two significant omissions. One is the clause which forbade the physician's use of surgery. Jones may be correct when he attributes this not to any Christian editing of the text but rather to the fact that, here also, the pagan text used by the Christian reviser did not itself include the clause. The second is the omission of the substantial section of the Oath which is addressed to the physician's relations with others in his profession – the closed circle of Hippocratic practice. Presumably the Christian reviser had no wish to establish a Christian guild of physicians along the lines of the original Hippocratics. This is one of a number of points at which the Christian version lacks the power of the original, and no doubt partly accounts for the fact that within Christendom it was the pagan form of the Oath which survived. This Christian version was left to gather dust in the libraries from which Dr Jones resurrected it.

Islamic Hippocratism

In clinical as opposed to ethical terms, the medical tradition of Greek antiquity was mediated to the mediaeval world largely through its adoption in Jewish and, especially, Arab medicine. There is growing awareness of the debt owed by the later Middle Ages to such Islamic scholars as Avicenna, and this is nowhere more true than in the medical field. What is of special interest to us is that this medicine was Hippocratic in character. Much of the extensive Hippocratic corpus was translated into Arabic, and the Oath with it. The same concern which led to the drafting of a Christian version of the Oath led also to its Islamicisation, in the process of translation, into a version which could be directly employed by Muslims. So in his study of *Islamic Medicine* Manfred Ullmann writes that, 'The fact that the Hippocratic Oath was demanded from the Arab doctors shows how strongly and for how long medical ethics were tied to his name.'[28]

In fact, the Islamic revision shows more sophistication than the Christian, and has been much more widely used. Aesculapius was historicised as the founder of medicine, and the particular characters of Hygeia and Panaceia were attributed to the Islamic God himself. So the Arabic Oath begins like this:

> I swear by God, Lord of life and death, the giver of health and the creator of healing and every therapy, and I swear by Asclepius and I swear by the saints of God, be they men or women, all together, and I appeal to them altogether as witnesses, that I shall stand by this oath and contract . . . [29]

The covenant form is here entirely preserved, even extended, and though re-sited in a different religious milieu, the Oath entirely retains its force. This testimony to the inherent adaptability of Hippocratism helps to explain its rapid spread through the ancient world and its tenacious hold on medicine in many different cultures even today.

Notes

1   This translation is as given by W. H. S. Jones in *The Doctor's Oath: an Essay in the History of Medicine*, Cambridge University Press, 1924, though Jones translates the names of Hygeia and Panaceia as Health and Heal-all; and I have added the headings. Some fluidity in the textual tradition is discussed below, though it does not seem to have left us with substantial uncertainties.

2   *Ibid.*, p. 46.

3   *Ibid.*, pp. 22f.

4   Oxford, 1978.

5   Jones, *The Doctor's Oath*, p. 39.

6   *Ibid.*, p. 40.

7   *Ibid.*

8   Danielle Gourévitch, *Le Triangle Hippocratique dans le Monde Greco–Romain*, Ecole Française de Rome, Rome, 1984.

9   Ludwig Edelstein, *The Hippocratic Oath. Text, Translation and Interpretation*, Johns Hopkins Press, Baltimore, 1943, p. vii.

10 *Ibid.*, p. 5.

11 *Ibid.*, p. 6.
12 *Ibid.*, p. 10.
13 *Ibid.*, p. 8. This often unrecognised facet of life in antiquity is given a very thorough examination by Danielle Gourevitch in *Le Triangle Hippocratique*, where a chart details much of our evidence for ancient medical suicides, achieved and contemplated.
14 Edelstein, *The Hippocratic Oath*, p. 9. A comparison with Gourévitch' survey is interesting (see note 13). Out of forty cases of medical suicide which she analyses, around one-quarter involved poison and as many again fasting, though the cause in other cases is not always evident.
15 *Ibid.*, p. 10.
16 *Ibid.*
17 *Ibid.*, pp. 12f.
18 *Ibid.*, p. 11.
19 *Ibid.*, p. 12.
20 *Ibid.*, p. 15.
21 *Ibid.*, pp. 16f.
22 *Ibid.*, p. 38. Edelstein goes on to offer a similar argument for the character of the covenant between teacher and pupil in which form the Oath is cast. He concludes: 'Not only the main feature of the covenant, the father–son relationship between teacher and pupil, but also all the detailed stipulations concerning the duties of the pupil can be paralleled by doctrines peculiar to the followers of Pythagoras. If related to Pythagoreanism, the specific formulas used in the covenant acquire meaning and definiteness.' *Ibid.*, p. 48.
23 *Ibid.*, p. 59. By 'medical deontology' all that is meant here is 'medical ethics'.
24 *Ibid.*, pp. 63f.
25 *Ibid.*, p. 64.
26 *Ibid.*, p. 59.
27 Jones, *The Doctor's Oath*, pp. 23ff.
28 M. Ullmann, *Islamic Medicine*, Edinburgh University Press, 1978, p. 11.
29 *Ibid.*, pp. 30f.

2

The Seamless Dress

What *is* medicine? That may seem a strange question to ask, but answers from doctors and medical students tend to show that those who practise medicine not only disagree about medical values, but that they also lack any single, unifying understanding of what it is they are doing.

Perhaps this criticism is unfair. Medical students are not taught in these terms. They are not invited to reflect systematically on the nature of medicine as a discipline but to practise it. If there are deficiencies in a system of medical education that fails to provoke in its students that kind of reflection, then there is a reason. This lies partly in increasing specialisation, partly in the rising profile of technology in medicine, partly in the break-up of the ethical consensus. The medical profession has simply forgotten to reflect on the nature of the medical enterprise. It has no single governing concept of what it is doing. A fatal combination of technological advance and ethical flux has led to the progressive disintegration of the idea of medicine.

To be fair, the combination of ethical flux and new technology has given rise to a remarkable growth in the discussion of medical ethics; from hospital ethics committees to government-sponsored reports as the basis for public policy. A parallel development in the academic world has led to the appointment of ethicists to university (and even hospital) staffs, though less so in the UK than in some other countries. Yet even in the USA, where legal and political factors have forced medical ethics into the front line of public concern, most medical education is carried on with only modest interest in 'bioethics'. And in the UK it is generally squeezed to the sidelines of the tightly packed medical curriculum. Although there is some interest in expanding this limited provision in the light of a spate of reports on medical–ethical issues and an avalanche of books, one effect has been to stress the variety of ethical options available to encourage an open-ended approach, and thus to hasten rather than slow the shift in values. Attention is focused on the challenge posed by new ethical options (especially as presented by new techniques), and there is little balancing interest in the values being displaced.

What is the clinician to make of all this? It leaves him confused, and rightly. In the smorgasbord of contemporary medical–ethical debate, there would seem to be something for everyone. In all its variety, contemporary medical–ethical discussion has the effect of offering him a prima facie ethical justification for whatever research or treatment regime he may happen to favour. The effective function of the bioethics enterprise – whatever individual writers and institutions may intend – is to offer ethical 'cover' for any and every proposed course of action. It is freedom from any specific ethical tradition – let alone that of Hippocratism – leaving bioethicists free to select whatever clinical option is favoured and, if they are so minded, to develop an appropriate apologia. To put it another way, there is no serious option in treatment or research which is entirely without an apologist in the field of academic bioethics.

Such an approach to contemporary discussion may seem cynical, but there is little public or professional (or political) awareness of the fact that the function of much current work in bioethics is entirely different from that which is traditionally associated with the word 'ethics' in medicine – the trying of practices and proposals in accordance with established principles of conduct. By contrast, a major role of the new bioethics has been to devise new principles of conduct which will allow practices which had hitherto been forbidden. There is no real analogy between the traditional 'ethical committees' of medical associations, which sit in judgment on professional conduct, or hospital 'ethical committees' which sift research proposals, and national ethical committees like the Warnock Committee in the UK and its equivalents worldwide.

These new bodies are established not to apply norms but to adjust them, and to draw up new ones if they wish. To say that is not to comment on the bona fide intentions of bioethicists, it is merely to set their endeavours in the context of the rapidly shifting values and uncertainty about fundamental norms which are the hallmark of these discussions in the 1980s and 1990s. The fact that some of the best-known figures in the bioethics world have defended extremely radical positions on substantive ethical issues is a much greater cause for alarm than is generally realised.

In this situation of conflict and confusion at the level of academic and public policy discussion, the working definitions of most medical practitioners are increasingly guided by two interlocking models of medicine, both of them deeply flawed: medicine as technique, and medicine as satisfaction of consumer wants.

The self-conscious introduction of an 'internal market' into the National Health Service in the UK illustrates this second model well, with its terminology of 'suppliers' and 'consumers' and its concept of health care as a commodity. Of course, most health care has always been privately supplied, and there is nothing necessarily bad about internal or open markets within health care systems (though market-led provision will undoubtedly accommodate faster ethical change and discriminate against certain classes such as the chronic sick). The dismay with which many have greeted these developments displays the threadbare character of our medicine, since there is little confidence that its ethics will hold up outside the state umbrella. The threads are hanging loose for all to see in the much freer market conditions of the USA. But the ethical character of Hippocratism has always precluded the reduction of health care provision into a mere market of consumer wants and health care providers.

This double model, with its conception of the physician as technician possessed of skills to dispense in the marketplace, is probably the inevitable concomitant of the abandonment of the ethical consensus. But it is nonetheless a threat, so much so that it raises the question whether medicine in this guise will survive. We return to this question in a later chapter, when we have surveyed some of the alternative ethical commitments which have been taken up into the new idea of medicine and which currently underlie growing areas of its practice. For the present we simply ask: thus defined and understood, would medicine ever have developed as it did? Would there ever have been the organic, professional development which gave birth to modern medicine? Are these ideas of medicine not the hallmarks of that very different medicine which existed before the Hippocratic revolution? That is to say, does not the contemporary breakdown of the ethical consensus, with its accompanying retreat into technique and consumerism, signal a return to the pre-Hippocratic norms?

THE NATURE OF HIPPOCRATIC MEDICINE

There is little appreciation of the truly extraordinary character of Hippocratic medicine. We have already noted Jones' complacent regard for the Hippocratic values as if, had Hippocrates not stated them, they would have emerged of their own accord as (in effect) self-evident. Jones could never have written that if he had been able to read some of the contemporary literature on medical ethics which is surveyed elsewhere in this book. The value of his comment is that it serves as an unconscious illustration of the degree to which, even as late as the first half of the twentieth century, the Hippocratic tradition had suffused western medicine. Hippocrates was so foundational that Jones found it impossible to conceive of any other kind of medicine.

It is strangely true that something which is taken for granted can be undermined with little conscious discussion of its merits. With the passage of time and the movement of opinion, the old tradition silently gives place to the new. In this case the evidence is striking in the paucity of literature on the subject. A computer library search is revealing in what it does *not* discover under the name of Hippocrates. And in the many general volumes which have been written on medicine, the lack of conscious reflection on the Hippocratic tradition is remarkable. Only very recently has Hippocrates been given more serious attention, and then as the target of critical comment from those who wish self-consciously to break with the tradition. Would-be defenders of Hippocrates have paid scant attention to what we have called the Hippocratic logic – the interplay of skills and moral commitments which make up the pattern of Hippocratic practice. At a time when flux and uncertainty in medicine have given rise to an unprecedentedly large volume of writing and publishing, it is strange that the name of Hippocrates should occur so rarely, and then almost invariably in formal, passing allusions.

It is not hard, of course, to find explanations for the contemporary writers' lack of enthusiasm for Hippocrates. There is plainly much in the Oath which cuts across contemporary *mores*, especially the Hippocratic perspective on the sanctity of life. By contrast, those who are most uneasy about abandoning Hippocratism have often failed to see the issue at stake in these terms. They have focused upon particular questions such as abortion, while it is the abandonment of Hippocratism itself which has prior significance. The final implications of departing from the tradition are of a different order altogether.

At the other end of the scale from Jones we have Ludwig Edelstein, who argued that since only a small minority of Greek physicians was sympathetic to Hippocratic values, the normative status claimed for them is groundless (however much we may happen to support them, as he did). One effect of his discussion was to give ammunition to those who would marginalise Hippocratic values, as is evident from the way in which his work was used by the US Supreme Court in the famous case of *Roe v. Wade*, which in 1973 liberalised the US law on abortion.

Though it had not been offered any arguments based upon the Oath, the Court itself raised the question in the course of a survey of historical attitudes to abortion. Edelstein's conclusion, that the Oath was a manifesto of the Pythagorean school and did not represent any general character in ancient medicine, gave the Court an opportunity to dismiss the relevance of traditional Hippocratic opposition to abortion. 'This, it seems to us, is a satisfactory and acceptable explanation of the Oath's apparent rigidity,'[1] wrote the Court, having cited Edelstein's remark that the Oath is 'a Pythagorean manifesto and not the expression of an absolute standard of medical conduct'.[2]

Yet, as we have already noted, Edelstein falls into the trap of false dichotomy. He may be correct in arguing the Pythagorean character of the Oath, but that has nothing to do with its validity. Indeed, as Edelstein had himself argued, the story of medicine in the years following the composition of the Oath is the story of the diffusion of its influence far beyond the bounds of the Pythagorean sect. The other so-called 'deontological' writings in the Hippocratic corpus (that is, those chiefly concerned with ethics rather than clinical practice) themselves reflect different philosophical milieux. Yet they exhibit a substantial harmony with the Oath, and, by their inclusion within the collection of books ascribed to Hippocrates, they show the enormous influence wielded by a medical tradition that had long since broken out of its Pythagorean confines. 'Among the general practitioners of late antiquity, the teaching of the deontological writings of the *Corpus Hippocraticum* seems to have prevailed.'[3]

The conquest of ancient medicine by Hippocratism, through its powerful blend of clinical expertise and moral ideas, cannot so easily be dismissed, as if something which began life as a 'Pythagorean manifesto' is therefore not 'an absolute standard of medical conduct'. Indeed, the Supreme Court itself speaks of the Oath as 'the apex of the development of strict ethical concepts in medicine'; and Edelstein himself stated, 'I trust that I am second to none in my appreciation of this document.'[4]

If we assume Edelstein's Pythagorean theory to be correct, the diffusion of Hippocratism throughout Greek medicine suggests that it fulfilled the ambitions of its originator. It is Edelstein himself who writes of the purpose of the Oath in the following terms: 'The Hippocratic Oath originally was a literary manifesto, a programme laid down by one who wished to set matters right in accordance with his own convictions.'[5]

The recognition that Hippocratism first emerged in ancient Greek society as a minority, reformist movement (which ultimately met with remarkable success) gives it new poignancy today. Its dominance of medicine is in question as it has never been since Hellenistic times. Hippocratism is in decline, once more the medical faith of a minority. In the process the Oath is returning to its original role – that of a manifesto for reform in medical values.

THE PROFESSION OF MEDICINE

We speak loosely of 'the medical profession' as if the phrase were merely a collective term for doctors. Yet it draws our attention to the professional character of medicine. Of course, there are other professions; and an assortment of occupations seeks to be added to their number, to indicate the freedom of its practitioners from the simple market reduction of the work to that of the tradesman. Teachers call themselves 'professionals', and we are now accustomed to speak of the 'teaching profession'; social workers are called 'professionals' too, though some would hesitate to call social work a 'profession', skilled and responsible though it be. What these uses of the term 'profession' suggest is that the idea is in the process of extension. To put it another way, these responsible occupations share some key aspects of what makes the old professions 'professions' – independence of judgment, confidentiality, round-the-clock commitment, and so forth. As traditionally understood, the 'professions' encompassed – alongside medicine – the law and, in a distinct sense, the Church. The profession was a vocation and its members were marked from the outset of their careers as the bearers of a characteristic set of responsibilities.

It is in this sense that medicine stands out as *the* profession, the profession *par excellence*. Even the other older professions, considered as professions, take their fundamental character from their analogy with medicine itself. It is in the values implied in Hippocratic medicine that we have the template of all professional commitment. In so far as other human occupations approximate to the professional character of Hippocratic medicine, they may be judged professions themselves. There is no bar to the analogical extension of the idea of the profession to education and social work, and much besides. By the same token, there is no bar to the withdrawal of this accolade from those whose concept or practice of their discipline does not share in the fundamental 'professional' character of Hippocratism.

It may be helpful at this point to refer to Edelstein's own discussion of the work of Scribonius Largus. Scribonius wrote at the beginning of the first century AD, so he gives us an opportunity to reflect on the character of medicine at the very outset of the Christian era, at a time when the influence of Hippocrates was already widely diffused in the ancient world. In his book *On Remedies* he writes of the 'sympathy' and 'humaneness' that arise from the 'will of medicine itself'. If the physician's heart is not full of these qualities, he will be despised by both gods and men. Scribonius goes on to spell out the obligations of the physician, who 'is not allowed to harm anybody, not even the enemies of the state . . . since medicine does not judge men by their circumstances in life, nor by their character. Rather does medicine promise her succor in equal measure to all who implore her help, and she professes never to be injurious to anyone.'[6] Scribonius goes on to refer to medicine as a 'profession' (*professio*). Edelstein comments: 'This word, in the language of his time, was applied to workmanship in preference to the older and morally indefinite terms, in order to emphasize the ethical connotations of work, the idea of an obligation or duty on the part of those engaged in the arts and crafts', among whom the physician was placed. He continues: 'It approximates most closely the Christian concept of "vocation" or "calling", except of course that for him who has been "called" to do a job his obligations are ordained by God, while for the member of an ancient profession his duties result from his own understanding of the nature of his profession.'[7]

This same concept underlies our modern idea of a profession, although in twentieth-century discussion there is more interest in the sociology of the profession than in the values which underlie it, and finally explain the social standing of physicians and the organisation of medicine in society. Thus one objective way of defining a profession over against other occupations is with regard to its self-regulating character, and the fact that it 'has assumed a dominant position in a division of labor, so that it gains control over the determination of the substance of its own work. Unlike most occupations, it is autonomous or self-directing.' We quote here from the Introduction to Eliot Freidson's *Profession of Medicine*, sub-titled 'A study in the sociology of applied knowledge'.

Freidson goes on to make a simple connection between the sociology of a profession and its values by seeking to account for its standing. 'The occupation sustains this special status by its persuasive profession of the extraordinary trustworthiness of its members,' a trustworthiness extending to both 'knowledgeable skill' and what Freidson calls 'ethicality'. And he continues:

The profession claims to be the most reliable authority on the nature of the reality it deals with. When its characteristic work lies in the attempt to deal with the problems people bring to it, the profession develops its own independent conception of those problems and tries to manage both clients and problems in its own way. In developing its own 'professional' approach, the profession changes the definition and shape of problems as experienced and interpreted by the layman. The layman's problem is re-created as it is managed – a new social reality is created by the profession. It is the autonomous position of the profession in society which enables it to re-create the layman's world.[8]

It is interesting to compare Freidson's discussion of the 'formal characteristics of a profession'. He notes that the fundamental distinction between a profession and other occupations 'lies in legitimate, organized autonomy . . . it has been given the right to control its own work'. Indeed, unlike any other occupation, Freidson makes the point that:

> . . . professions are *deliberately* granted autonomy, including the exclusive right to determine who can legitimately do its work and how the work should be done. Virtually all occupations struggle to obtain both rights, and some manage to seize them, but only the profession is *granted* the right to exercise them legitimately. And while no occupation can prevent employers, customers, clients, and other workers from evaluating its work, only the profession has the recognized right to declare such 'outside' evaluation illegitimate and intolerable.[9]

But if this remarkable autonomous status is a mark of the medical profession above all others, who grants it? Freidson observes that 'it is unlikely that one occupation would be chosen spontaneously over others and granted the singular status of a profession by some kind of popular vote. Medicine was certainly not so chosen. A profession attains and maintains its position by virtue of the protection and patronage of some elite segment of society which has been persuaded that there is some special value in its work.'

And Freidson continues by drawing attention to the reason why, in a high civilisation, the 'elite segment' should treat a profession in this manner:

> The work of the chosen occupation is unlikely to have been singled

out if it did not represent or express some of the important beliefs or values of that elite . . . the work of the profession needs have no necessary relationship to the beliefs or values of the average citizen. But once a profession is established in its protected position of autonomy, it is likely to have a dynamic of its own . . . The work of the profession may thus eventually diverge from that expected by the elite . . . It is essential for survival that the dominant elite remain persuaded of the positive values, or at least the harmlessness, of the profession's work, so that it continues to protect it from encroachment.[10]

There are notable parallels between Freidson's analysis and ours, in respect of the nature of a profession and its relations with the society which through its elite accords it its status, and whose beliefs and values, as focused in those of the elite, it represents. Freidson's discussion of the need for and problem of professional survival is particularly illuminating. The threat of divergence between professional beliefs and values and those of the elite is serious, since it would undermine the standing of the profession in society. If medicine is unable to ensure that the 'dominant elite remain persuaded' of its values and task, it is open to the profession to shift the emphases of values and task alike in order that they might approximate the more closely with those acceptable to the elite. Of course, this would not be – has not been – a conscious ploy, since the leaders of the profession, who set the key of its self-understanding, are in contemporary society themselves members of the elite. Medicine is not quite a monastic exercise. It is closed but not impervious, autonomous yet not entirely isolated from the value-system of the society in which its own values are traded.

To some extent this is the price which the profession has paid for its very 'professional' status, in Freidson's terms. It has gained a unique recognition from society's elite, but in so doing has altogether lost any consciousness that its values were once 'peculiarly those of a small and isolated group' which had gathered around a radical and reforming 'manifesto'.[11] Ironically, it was in so doing that it played a major part in the development of the very idea of a profession.

We return to a number of Freidson's observations in due course. For the present, suffice it to note that in the nascent

Hippocratic medicine of the ancient world we have the emergence of the physician's art as a professional enterprise. It is not merely that; indeed, the other historic professions of the law and the Church are in important respects distinct from medicine, such that to speak of the 'idea of a profession' can be misleading. We do better to recognise that this idea is always relative to the particular character of the profession concerned. Some general observations may be made, along the lines of those we have cited from Freidson. Yet even they have a special application to medicine rather than to other professions, ancient or modern. It is interesting to note that while his study is of medicine, it is intended to be of medicine as an example, *the* example, of the character of a profession. So, in Freidson's own words, medicine is 'not merely one of the major professions of our time . . . Indeed, in one way or another, the profession of medicine, not that of law or the ministry or any other, has come to be the prototype upon which occupations seeking a privileged status today are modelling their aspirations.'[12]

We have already suggested such a status for medicine, arising from the suffusion of the medical enterprise with moral commitments. We have also suggested that, historically, the beginnings of the idea of a profession may be traced to the rise of Hippocratism in medicine, though that is not to exclude other sources, Christian and pagan, from such a packaging of virtue and skill in society. What it does is to draw attention to the character of medicine as *the* profession. In his own analysis Freidson, like other modern writers on medicine as a profession, exaggerates the significance of those factors which have changed the character of medical practice down the centuries. From the perspective of those whose interest in medicine as a profession is sociological rather than ethical this may be inevitable, but in dividing modern medicine from its ancient progenitor such an approach fails to grasp the moral logic of Hippocratism, which gave birth to the western medical tradition, and which today still underlies medicine in its professional character.

MEDICINE AS MORAL COMMITMENT

The question which such a discussion inevitably raises is that of the inner character of medicine. How is it to be understood, in its essentials? Is modern medicine in real continuity with ancient practice – and, therefore, with medical practice today in primitive situations, where both modern techniques and the structure of the consulting and autonomous profession are absent? Freidson goes so far as to indicate the later part of the nineteenth century as the period when medicine developed as a profession, in the sense which most interests him. Yet such an abstraction arises out of the field of interest of the sociologist, rather than the medical tradition itself. We must ask why medicine has developed as a marriage of skill and moral commitment, why it emerged in antiquity as a principled and philanthropic enterprise. The origins of the idea of medicine as a profession lie in the particular set of moral commitments which have from the start constituted the Hippocratic tradition.

The character of medicine as moral commitment has been nowhere better expressed than by Stanley Hauerwas, especially in his essays collected in the volume *Suffering Presence*, where he gives free rein to his thinking on a spread of topics which intersect with the question of medicine and the handicapped.[13] He draws attention to the growing popularity of medical ethics. 'Confronted by issues that seemed morally troubling,' he writes, 'physicians began to acknowledge that medicine must again touch base with ethics.' Yet 'as a result, many failed to notice that medicine was first and foremost a moral practice constituted by intrinsic moral convictions that are operative even if not explicitly acknowledged.'[14]

As we have argued, the moral convictions which Hauerwas here suggests are intrinsic to medicine were, in fact, acknowledged most explicitly in the Hippocratic Oath. The Hippocratic physician lays his cards on the table; or, in terms of the Oath itself, before commencing his medical studies the would-be Hippocratic doctor picks up a set of moral cards at the outset. He knows, and his patients know, what his teacher, in passing on the tradition, insists: that the moral commitments of the physician are of the essence of medical practice. They are not some added extra, optional and a matter of preference. They are integral to the practice of the profession, to its very professional character. Of course, there were physicians before Hippocrates. But (and this is the point lying behind Hauerwas' statement) they were not practising what we have come to mean by medicine. At the heart of Hippocratism lies the conviction that medical values are intrinsic and not extrinsic to the medical enterprise. The plainest and most disturbing feature of contemporary medical–ethical discussion is the readiness with which even those who share the substantive values of the tradition are falling victim to the claim that these are mere super-additions to the technique which characterises and determines the nature of medicine. Most physicians, at least, remain men and women of integrity, working within the framework of their own moral convictions. But, in their view, the heart of medicine is not moral commitment, however important personal and particular moral commitments may be. Medicine is technique.

The attraction of such a view of the essence of medicine is obvious. It enables those who wish to break with the moral tradition of Hippocrates to maintain their claim to be practising that same 'art' of which he was an exponent. They have merely shuffled the pack of moral cards. They maintain that Hippocratic values are subjective, arbitrary, claiming the opposite of Jones' unintentionally disparaging notion that they are really self-evident. They are time-bound, and bound also by particular religious and philosophical commitments. This was in essence the case of the US Supreme Court against the claims of the Hippocratic tradition in *Roe v. Wade*. Taking Edelstein's analysis as their point of departure, they moved on to relativise the moral commitments of Hippocratism as merely those of Pythagorean physicians in ancient Greece. There is no interest shown in the extraordinary Hippocratic marriage of value and technique which gave rise to the development of western medicine. Its implications for the significance of these 'merely' Pythagorean values seems to have escaped critics of the tradition. In current debate, this view is typical, and it enables contemporary apologists for the new medicine to lay claim to continuity with the old.

Of course they cannot altogether escape the overweening influence of Hippocratism. Every one of the modern re-statements of medical values has unconsciously or (generally) consciously cast itself in the Hippocratic form. The claim to stand within the great tradition of the old medicine is all but universal. Yet it is a claim which increasingly lacks credibility; the continuity is one of form, and can be claimed only by manipulating the substance of the tradition. The historical character of Hippocratism as a dissident, reforming movement which integrated clinical skill and distinct moral commitment gives the lie to such a claim.

What then is the nature of the Hippocratic tradition? Out of what inner logic is woven its seamless dress? We have surveyed the text of the Oath and its history, and referred to the many contemporary versions which it has spawned in the twentieth century. It remains for us to gain a perspective on Hippocratism as a whole. The origins of modern medicine lie in the extraordinary moral power of the Hippocratic Oath and the ancient tradition which it represents. This conviction depends no more on the 'legend' of Hippocrates of Cos than upon the historical reconstruction of Ludwig Edelstein in his monograph of 1943.

There is no doubt that in Hippocratism we see the emergence in late Greek antiquity of a tightly knit body of moral thinking as the Siamese twin of effective clinical practice. If the 'legend' had graduates of ancient medical schools raising their right arm and swearing the Oath in full academic dress, it may be discounted with no loss. More exhilarating is Edelstein's realistic reconstruction of a vigorous, reforming minority, stemming from the disciples of later Pythagoreanism but soon diffusing into one philosophical school after another, until finally the legend could be written and believed. This analysis suggests a remarkable demonstration of the power of an idea. With the spread of Christianity throughout the Graeco–Roman world, the idea's time had come. Its ethics – as demanding as those of the Pythagoreans – could be undergirt with a theology of grace, and its moral power, already widely diffused in the different philosophical strands of the medicine of late antiquity, could be harnessed by the Christian Church. Its influence even on post-Christian western medicine, struggling to free and re-establish itself as a secular enterprise, testifies to its enduring power and the degree to which the warp and woof of medical values and skills are interwoven in the Hippocratic fabric.

The starting point of the tradition, first pagan and then baptised into Christian service, lies in its conviction that the physician is a healer. This underlies the scope of the Hippocratic enterprise. We may take that for granted, but its significance emerges in the prohibitions of the Oath which have so plainly stamped the Hippocratic tradition, ancient as modern, with the character of a healing tradition, pure and simple.

Hippocratism is healing and not harming. The famous medical principle *primum non nocere* (first, or above all, do no harm) is to be found not in the Oath itself but elsewhere in the body of Hippocratic writings. Yet it could as well have been in the Oath, since it is in the Oath that the two fundamental medical 'harms' are spelled out – together with the other more general harms in the power of the unscrupulous physician.

The prohibition of the medical harms, more than all else, sets the practice of Hippocratism apart from that of any other kind of medicine. For they are harms which might be done as readily by the scrupulous as by the unscrupulous, by the man of integrity as by the rogue. Their prohibition is the badge of the medical ethics of Hippocratism, as opposed to its medical etiquette. These harms are those of abortion and euthanasia. The Hippocratic physician forswears them. To be more precise, in the terms of the Oath – whether or not it was ever employed in such a fashion – the medical student, before taking up his studies, binds himself irrevocably to a medical practice which excludes participation in the taking of human life, before birth or after. And (in the formal stipulations of the Oath, which are intended to govern the passing on of medical knowledge) he will impart none of his expertise to any who will not swear likewise. The medical arts, whose supreme clinical, as well as ethical, manifestation in ancient times was found in Hippocrates, could be revealed only to those who would hold these two together.

It is in this clear, though negative, definition of the limits of the healer's task that we find the Hippocratic avowal of the principle of the sanctity of human life. The negative form which it takes is plainly deliberate. In place of a doctrine about the nature of human life we find practical provisions designed to protect it.

As we have already noted, the precise form of the prohibitions stands for a broader restriction on the practice of the physician. Abortions were procured in the ancient world by a variety of means. Apparently the most common method used a pessary. By the same token, suicides for medical reasons – not uncommon, we read – could of course be brought about in many different ways. But the administration of poison, either by the physician himself or by the patient, was the most usual; and although poisons were generally available, it was evidently normal for the physician himself to supply an appropriate remedy. Since suicide–euthanasia and abortion were widespread in the Graeco–Roman world, and since the physician was generally involved in both of them, the distinctive and radical character of Hippocratism is revealed in sharp focus as would-be arbiter of the ethics of the profession. A new and uncompromising moral agenda was set for medical practice.

Though these twin negations form the most significant clauses to be found in the Oath, they are to be balanced against its most significant omission. It comes as a surprise to many people – not least, to physicians – to realise that the Oath makes no specific reference among the responsibilities of the doctor to the relief of human suffering. This is plainly intended to underline the Hippocratic opposition to abortion and euthanasia, since their defence lay – as it lies today – in a relief-of-suffering ethic devoid of a commitment to the sanctity of human life. In ancient Greece, even more than today, the palliative role of the physician would have been central. Clinical management options would have been few – in a primitive culture where drug therapies and surgery were severely limited, and long before the development of antisepsis and anaesthesia. The physician often must have faced no alternative to whatever palliative means lay at his disposal. Yet the Oath makes no reference to what for many physicians today would have pride of place in their ordering of medical commitments: while the prohibition of abortion and suicide–euthanasia is underlined, the duty to relieve suffering is left unmentioned. So what is the key to the moral medicine of Hippocrates?

We turn back now to the Oath to seek an understanding of the structure of the moral and religious commitments involved in Hippocratism. The first thing which strikes us is its sophistication: it is very far from the simplistic medical creed which some of its contemporary critics imply. There are different ways in which the Oath and its moral structure could be analysed. In the remainder of this chapter we draw out three interlocking principles which together determine the Hippocratic logic. Firstly, we examine its triple covenantal character, in which the physician is covenanted to his God, his master and his patient. Secondly, we turn to the double ethical principle which, within this multiple covenant, governs the physician's practice of his profession: a due regard for the sanctity of human life, and a general philanthropy in which his patient's interests are always paramount. Thirdly, we focus on the single role of the Hippocratic physician: he is a healer.

The Triple Covenant

We suggested in our discussion of the ancient Christian version of the Oath that the excision of most of the covenantal features was a major impoverishment. The displacement of its covenantal structure leaves the Oath a naked ethical code, while its moral force depends precisely upon its being more than that. Other revisions have tended to have the same effect, though in almost every post-Hippocratic code there are the remnants of the original covenantal structure. The structure itself is highly complex.

We may outline it as follows. The pupil/physician who swears the Oath commits himself to much more than a code of practice. For the logic of that practice arises from a series of relationships. Chiefly they are three in number, though a fourth is referred to and others are implied.

The physician stands in covenantal relationship to his master, who has inducted him into the medical arts (and also to his master's family); to his patient; and to his God, before whom he sets the whole conduct of his medical vocation, as of his life. There is reference also to those who will in due time be his own pupils, in the solemn promise to impart medical instruction only to those who have already committed themselves to the Hippocratic values. This represents an adjunct to his covenant with his teacher, who is thereby assured that what he has imparted to his pupil will never be passed on, except on the same terms – to one who, like his pupil, stands in the closed Hippocratic circle.

The implied relationships are themselves interesting, since just as the master shares a responsible concern for future pupils of the one whom he has taught, so he has a concern for his student's patients; indeed, it is out of this concern that the tradition is to be strictly maintained. Moreover, in swearing the Oath the physician is acknowledging that in his treatment of his patients he is treating those for whom he is accountable to God. The physician's God has his own interest in the physician's patients.

All of which underlines the complex nexus of covenant to which the Hippocratic physician commits himself by oath. His practice of medicine, and the moral commitments which underlie it, are no private matters in which he acts alone. The medical vocation draws him into a set of relationships which make fundamental demands on him and determine the character of the medical practice in which he engages. They oblige him, in turn, to pass on his clinical skills only to those who will first submit to the self-same covenantal ethical context. This is no self-seeking closed shop of a medical guild, as has sometimes been suggested; it is fundamental to the moral character of the tradition: only by refusing to pass on the medical arts to those outside the ambit of its values can the Hippocratic physician demonstrate his own moral seriousness. Here is a clear initiation of a medical–moral tradition: it is built into this understanding of the physician's responsibility to his teacher and his pupil, as well as his patient. It is in the nature of Hippocratism that it makes no claim to be merely sectional, or indeed sectarian. Its claim is objective, to represent the truth about human nature and to deny all other possible understandings as untrue. The exclusivity of the Hippocratic tradition is the result, and has been no small contributor to its influence.

We look in a later chapter at the significance for medicine of a covenantal understanding of the doctor–patient relationship. As we shall see, this key concept has been recognised in contemporary debate, though it has not commended itself universally. Yet its grounding in this Hippocratic three-way covenant is not recognised. The vertical reference of the Oath – to God – is in both Pythagorean and Christian conceptions of medicine the crucial context of the human relationships involved. Otherwise the Oath, like some of its secular revisions, would present a mere formal code, a cold set of rules. By contrast, Hippocratic ethics are theistic. We have suggested that they might even be described as theological ethics, in however rudimentary a form.

The human covenants are grounded in a divine covenant; the human obligations in obligations to God. That, of course, is the source of the self-confidence which gives rise to the claim of Hippocratic exclusivity. The Hippocratic physician is in no position to negotiate his ethical perceptions; he must do nothing which will encourage the development of clinical practice outside of the very special covenantal context in which he has been led to practise. This is not simply because he has so promised his teacher, or because he personally believes such practice to be wrong. It is because he has so promised his God, and he is convinced that Hippocratism is the only basis on which his God would have him engage in the medical enterprise. The exclusivity of such a position is but the corollary of its internal logic.

In Chapter One we commented briefly on the contents of the Oath. What needs to be added is the broader perspective in which these individual commitments and injunctions should be understood. We must be grateful to Edelstein for the light which his work has thrown on the origins of Hippocratism in the Pythagoreanism of the later fourth century BC. We here add to our debt, since Edelstein's own argument demonstrates that the values of the Oath represent the outworking in the field of medicine of certain specific religious–philosophical convictions. The Hippocratic physicians swear their Oath before God since it represents the sum of what they believe he demands of them as physicians. The interlocking of the human and divine covenants is not arbitrary. In no other way could a 'pure and holy' life be lived, or a 'pure and holy' art practised. Because of the theistic grounding of the ethical injunctions of the Oath, the covenantal obligations to teacher, patient and God come to a single focus.

The Two-fold Obligation

We can sum up the ethical character of the Oath in the twin obligations of philanthropy and the sanctity of life. As we have noted, each of these could be held to entail the other. Yet it is convenient to distinguish those injunctions in the Oath which expressly forbid the taking of life from those in which the physician is enjoined to seek the well-being of his patient – and nothing else. It appears at first as if these represent the negative and the positive, in order to leave no room at all for doubt as to the character of the conduct required of the physician. In fact we see in the negative aspects of the Oath's moral injunctions (as in the Ten Commandments) sophistication that is born of realism. Hippocratism is no mere lofty ideal. We may well believe with Jones that the Oath (even in some earlier form) must surely have an historical connection with Hippocrates of Cos. He was no ivory tower ethicist but the greatest clinician in the ancient world.

But we note here that just as such questions as confidentiality and sexual continence are addressed directly and by prohibition, so is the sanctity of human life. In fact the Oath says nothing about the sanctity of life in so many words, it simply outlaws any participation in its destruction. In this respect there is a notable contrast between the Oath and some of its contemporary restatements, which focus on positive rather than negative viewpoints and thereby leave open possibilities of qualification and reinterpretation. Had the Declaration of Geneva followed the Oath in banning abortion instead of opting for a positive alternative statement, which had the same intention – 'utmost respect . . . from the time of conception' – it would have been altogether more difficult to slip gears into ambiguity and revise the text, when liberal abortion was on the horizon, to read ' . . . from its beginning'. We return to this in Chapter Three.

The Single Role

It seems mere tautology to suggest that the role of the Hippocratic physician is that of a healer, but it puts some of the most contentious issues in contemporary medical–ethical debate into focus. Indeed, there is no more concise way of drawing attention to the contrast between the old medicine and the new. The anguish of contemporary medicine is that it finds itself locked in a conflict between the Hippocratic model of the healer and the attempt to set in his place a new physician whose chief task is to 'relieve suffering'. The dialectic of healing and the relief of suffering is the crucible of the new medicine; but it was also the crucible of the old.

That is a fact of central importance in any attempt to assess the relevance of Hippocratic values today. As we have seen in our discussion of the historical origins of the Hippocratic tradition, at a series of key points – and especially in its opposition to both abortion and suicide–euthanasia — Hippocratism consciously defined itself over against the contemporary medical *mores* of antiquity in which the 'relief of suffering' had pride of place. This is not, of course, the whole story; and the reforming Hippocratic manifesto had also set its sights on other abuses. But in repudiating both abortion and suicide–euthanasia, the Hippocratic physicians defiantly rejected a relief-of-suffering ethic, setting in its place the ethic which we know by the name of the sanctity of life.

The effect of ruling out these options, and especially that of euthanasia, is to channel the medical enterprise in one direction, and one only. Medicine becomes synonymous with healing, and forswears absolutely the option of taking human life. To prevent all possible misunderstanding this conviction is underlined by the strangest of all omissions from the Oath. As we have already noted, many medical practitioners are astonished to learn that the Oath says nothing explicit about the calling of the physician to relieve the suffering of his patients. Of course, philanthropy runs right through the Oath. But in this regard its implications are not specified. Since this document details the calling and principles of the physician so fully, it is impossible to avoid the conclusion that there is a reason why 'relieving suffering' remains undiscussed. In the Oath itself we see recognition of the danger posed by the relief-of-suffering ethic, subversive as it is of the very Hippocratic idea, short-circuiting the healing task by putting the patient's life under threat from the doctor himself.

Even so, perhaps some reference could have been made to relieving suffering as a subordinate task, secondary to the healing role of the physician. The omission is heavy with significance. Here, as in other matters, the Oath is characterised by a caution which speaks to our contemporary situation. For today we see what Hippocrates witnessed in Greek antiquity: a medicine in which healing is not paramount. Of course, healing remains *an* objective of the physician, but only if it seems the best way of 'relieving suffering'. For Hippocrates, the relief of suffering is incidental, assumed in the commitment to secure the patient's general well-being. Far from being merely semantic, this difference is profound, the touchstone of a medical tradition, the watershed in antiquity and the modern world between Hippocratism and primitive, pre-Hippocratic medicine.

The single-minded character of the Hippocratic healing commitment has successfully protected western medicine from the unresolved, double-minded tensions of a medical tradition in which both healing and the 'relief of suffering' vie for status. Yet this is how many physicians today understand their task, as a balancing act between the two in which, in every case, a fresh framework of understanding requires to be established. The result is to set at the heart of clinical practice an illogic which seems to deny any single mission for medicine. The tendency is to give way to those pressures which have displaced healing from its paramount position in the tradition and to subsume it beneath the 'relief of suffering'. The physician may actually believe that he is working with two equal principles, while in practice subordinating healing to 'relief' on every single occasion – since, whenever they come into conflict, the one takes precedence over the other. We return to this theme in a later chapter.

Notes

1   410 US 116 (1973).
2   Ludwig Edelstein, *The Hippocratic Oath*, p. 64.
3   Ludwig Edelstein, 'The Professional Ethics of the Greek Physician', in *Bulletin of the History of Medicine* 30 (1956), pp. 392–418; repr. in S. J. Reiser, A. J. Dyck, W. J. Curran, edd., *Ethics in Medicine: Historical Perspectives and Contemporary Concerns*, MIT Press, Cambridge, Mass. and London, 1983, p. 46.
4   *Ibid.*, p. 42.
5   *Ibid.*, p. 43.
6   *Ibid.*, pp. 44f.
7   *Ibid.*, p. 45. Edelstein goes on to contrast this 'ideal of medical humanism' with the 'spirit of Hippocratic ethics', suggesting that even Scribonius could make the connection only 'by implication'. But Scribonius, who called Hippocrates 'the father

of our profession', plainly believed himself to be unpacking Hippocratic values.

8   Eliot Freidson, *Profession of Medicine: a Study in the Sociology of Applied Knowledge*, Harper & Row, New York, 1970, p. xvii.
9   *Ibid.*, pp. 71f.
10   *Ibid.*, pp. 72f.
11   Edelstein, *The Hippocratic Oath*, p. 38.
12   Freidson, *Profession of Medicine*, p. xviii.
13   Stanley Hauerwas, *Suffering Presence*, University of Notre Dame Press, Indiana, 1986; T. & T. Clark, Edinburgh, 1988.
14   *Ibid.*, p. 4.

3

Germany and Geneva: Challenge and Response

This chapter may seem a curious diversion. Yet we cannot ignore the single, stark occasion in the western medical tradition when the profession turned its back on the Hippocratic legacy. The context of the 'medical crimes' which were tried at Nuremberg was that of an unique political situation in which many leading elements of German society were deeply corrupted. Is it surprising that doctors were corrupted too? Yet that simply underlines the extraordinary nature of the episode. As we have seen, medicine as a profession is closely related to the ruling elite in any society. The medical profession is liable to follow any fundamental shift in society's values. What is remarkable and alarming is the rapidity with which German medicine submitted to the political dictates of the Nazi regime and, moreover, the contribution which discussions within medicine played in assisting in their execution. Resistance on the part of the German medical profession was lamentably limited.

We can go so far as to say that in the light of the conservative character of medicine, and the self-consciously traditional values which it has espoused, the rapid collapse of German medical ethics in the 1930s suggests that Hippocratic values are far more vulnerable than might have been thought possible, although it is evident that the process had begun some time before the rise of National Socialism in German politics. These developments present the alarming prospect of medical values in free fall.

Much has been written in recent years about the developments in German medicine which foreshadowed the experience of the Second World War and the immediate post-war years – the institution of euthanasia, and then the barbarity of medicine in the death camps. We can sketch this background before we go on to summarise these two sorry chapters in western medical history. Then we survey the response which they elicited in the desire of the post-war medical community to re-affirm its Hippocratic lineage. That response offers adequate justification for this chapter, since it is not widely realised that the context of the Declaration of Geneva is Nazi medicine. The fact that the World Medical Association found it necessary to re-state its values in this manner requires us to take medicine under the Third Reich seriously *as medicine*, and not simply as an excrescence of Nazi ideology.

The judgment of the international medical community was that in the aftermath of war it had no alternative but to re-affirm its identity. The World Medical Association saw what had happened to German medicine under the Third Reich as a betrayal of the Hippocratic tradition. West Germany's generally conservative stance in subsequent bioethical discussion – in the development of *in vitro* technology, abortion, attitudes to euthanasia – is the echo of an anguished conscience.

The explanation of such lingering post-war concern is that the point of contact between German medicine then and now does not lie in the barbarism of the camps. That was indeed the nadir of Hippocratism, but because it was also the consequence of a complex of opportunism, political ideology and the numbing experience of warfare, its betrayal of the medical tradition was only at one remove. The signal point of departure from the humane tradition of western medicine lies in the euthanasia programme with which pre-war Germany busied itself, exterminating its own citizens and beginning with mentally defective children.

These events were not the cause of what followed; indeed, they shared a common cause in the intellectual developments which precipitated Nazi ideology. Yet few would deny that what happened in pre-war German medicine helped prepare the way for the atrocities of the camps. The German medical profession did not resist the euthanasia programme. And the fact that it was unresisting, aside from illustrating the fascination which National Socialism held for so much of German society, aided its acquiescence in what was to follow. The euthanasia programme marked the point at which German medicine withdrew from many centuries of western Hippocratic consensus.

In fact, the relationship between National Socialist ideology and German medical tradition during the inter-war period is complex. A key role was played by the 'race-hygiene' movement in pre-Nazi Germany which, with its origins in the international development of social Darwinism at the turn of the century, led in Germany to the dominance of a brand of eugenics which became increasingly racialist in character.[1] Side by side there was growing debate about euthanasia, not merely in Germany but throughout the West. In Germany itself a most influential book was *Release and Destruction of Lives not Worth Living* by Alfred Hoche and Rudolph Binding, published in 1920. But already German medicine and the body politic had begun to part company with the Hippocratic consensus. This famous book appeared in the immediate aftermath of the First World War. During that war nearly half of all patients in German mental hospitals had died of starvation or disease. At a time of national shortages they merited a low priority.[2]

One of the most disturbing of recent studies was translated into English as *Murderous Science*. Its author, Benno Müller-Hill, is currently Professor of Genetics in the University of Cologne. By way of introduction to his account of the corruption of German science, he offers a chronological summary of major events before and during the war years. The events he lists include the following:

14 July 1933 [only five and a half months after Hitler became Chancellor] The 'law for the prevention of progeny with hereditary defects' is proclaimed. It allows for compulsory sterilization in cases of 'congenital mental defects, schizophrenia, manic-depressive psychosis, hereditary epilepsy . . . and severe alcoholism'.

Spring 1937 A decision is made that all German coloured children are to be illegally sterilized. After the prerequisite expert reports are provided by Dr Abel, Dr Schade, and Professor Fischer, the sterilizations are carried out.[3]

THE EUTHANASIA PROGRAMME

Müller-Hill's summary continues:

24 March 1938 Professor Kleist, a psychiatrist . . . report[s] on the mental hospital in Herborn, where euthanasia by starvation was being practised . . .

1 September 1939 With his assault on Poland Hitler begins the Second World War. He backdates his letter introducing 'euthanasia' to the same date: 'Reichsleiter Bouhler and Dr Brandt are entrusted with the responsibility of extending the rights of specially designated physicians, such that patients who are judged incurable after the most thorough review of their condition which is possible can be granted mercy killing.'

October 1939 Following these instructions, the first question-naires are distributed to mental hospitals. They are completed by . . . [nine] professors of psychiatry, and thirty-nine other doctors of medicine. Their payment is 5 pfennigs per questionnaire, when more than 3500 are processed per month, up to 10 pfennigs when there are less than 500. A cross signifies death. There are 283 000 questionnaires to be processed. These experts mark at least 75 000 with a cross.[4]

It is important to realise that the programme was compulsory only for the patients – not for participating physicians. 'Doctors were never ordered to murder psychiatric patients and handicapped children. They were empowered to do so, and fulfilled their task without protest, often on their own initiative.' Indeed, 'the killings were performed contrary to German law, though authorized by government officials.'[5] This fact is underlined by the evidence that charges of murder were actually brought against the heads of institutions after parents' complaints that they believed their children to have been killed; though they were dropped when the courts were informed that Hitler had granted immunity to those involved.[6] Various steps were taken to counter parental and other public opposition – some parents were deprived of custody of their children, and others were themselves arrested.[7]

Yet despite spasmodic parental protest, there was a remarkable unanimity among the professionals involved in this process. Müller-Hill writes: 'As far as the anthropologists and human geneticists were concerned, I believe that I can say with certainty that none differed in any important respect from those whom I have named.' Much the same could be said of psychiatrists. Only a handful of individuals are known to have protested, or even to have stood aside from the process. Some others sought a softening of the programme, voicing concern about its legality or the public disquiet which it had engendered; but the fact that they participated simply gave added force to the underlying principles of the programme, which they were unable or unwilling to question. Müller-Hill concludes:

I know no written testimony against euthanasia from a psychiatrist. Ernst Klee, who has studied all the records connected with euthanasia prosecutions, names one psychiatrist in a mental hospital, Dr H. Jasperson, who denounced the euthanasia programme, and who tried in vain to persuade the heads of the university departments of psychiatry to make a collective protest. I know of no psychiatrist who was suspended or dismissed because of such a protest.

He adds: 'No German psychiatrist accompanied his patients on their last journey. There were no martyrs.' We may compare Proctor's chilling conclusion: 'The record of medicine under the Nazis is largely one of eager and active cooperation; and neither resistance nor indifference was able to offset the enthusiasm of the profession for the regime and its policies.'[8]

It is worth noting that this final solution to the problem of the mentally ill has its origins in their general abuse in German psychiatric institutions. This goes back to the First World War and looks forward to the concentration camps. Müller-Hill writes that:

The provincial psychiatric hospitals had become custodial institutions in which the patients waited, without treatment, either for death or for discharge . . . From the 1920s onwards, the introduction of unpaid forced labour ('work-therapy') made these institutions important from an economic point of view too . . . The psychiatric institutions were very much like the concentration camps.[9]

The connection with the rise of 'race-hygiene' thinking is clear: it reversed the tradition of humane treatment of the sick and defective by casting them in the new role of a threat to the race.

Leo Alexander, in an influential and recently reprinted article first published in the 1949 *New England Journal of Medicine*, set these developments in context for readers who had only just discovered the full story of what Alexander called 'Medical Science under Dictatorship'. Alexander was a psychiatrist who had worked with the prosecuting counsel in the Nuremberg medical trials. He outlined the story in stark terms, and acknowledged that though 'Nazi propaganda was highly effective in perverting public opinion and public conscience', leading to 'a rapid decline in standards of professional ethics', the roots lay deeper than in the phenomenon of the Nazi dictatorship itself. To that extent his title was misleading, and could distract attention from developments internal to the medical profession which were congruent with, and amenable to, pressure from political ideology outside.[10] Müller-Hill points out that these developments were unique to Germany. They had no parallel in the Fascism of Spain or Italy.

Alexander writes:

> Even before the Nazis took open charge in Germany, a propaganda barrage was directed against the traditional compassionate nineteenth-century attitudes toward the chronically ill, and for the adoption of a utilitarian, Hegelian point of view. Sterilization and euthanasia of persons with chronic mental illnesses was discussed at a meeting of Bavarian psychiatrists in 1931. By 1936 extermination of the physically or socially unfit was so openly accepted that its practice was mentioned incidentally in an article published in an official German medical journal.[11]

Alexander then instances two telling examples of propaganda designed to influence public attitudes to the euthanasia programme:

Adults were propagandized by motion pictures, one of which, entitled 'I Accuse' deals entirely with euthanasia. This film depicts the life history of a woman suffering from multiple sclerosis; in it her husband, a doctor, finally kills her to the accompaniment of soft piano music rendered by a sympathetic colleague in an adjoining room. Acceptance of this ideology was implanted even in the children. A widely-used high-school mathematics text . . . includes problems stated in distorted terms of the cost of caring for and rehabilitating the chronically sick and crippled.[12]

In the one-sentence letter we quoted (see p. 72), Hitler formally announced the euthanasia programme at the beginning of the war. Brandt and Bouhler set about their work with enthusiasm. The questionnaires to which we have already referred required state mental institutions to report on inmates who had been ill for five years or more and who were unable to work. Alexander translates the name of the committee which evaluated these returns as the Reich 'Work Committee for Institutions for Cure and Care'. At the same time, to ensure that the institutions thus emptied would not begin to refill, a second organisation was established specifically to deal with the problem posed by children. The 'Reich Commission for the Registration of Severe Disorders in Childhood' was set up, consisting of paediatricians, to establish euthanasia criteria for children and to deal with individual cases. During 1939 and 1940 its work was limited to handicapped newborns and children under the age of four. Later on it turned its attention also to the killing of adolescents.[13]

Outside Germany itself there was less concern for formalities. One SS chief could write to Himmler as follows (in January 1940):

The other two units of storm troopers at my disposal were employed as follows during October, November and December . . . For the elimination of about 4400 incurable patients from Polish mental hospitals . . . For the elimination of about 2000 incurable patients from the Konradstein mental hospital . . .[14]

The same approach was taken with mental institutions further east, whose inmates were shot as the German armies moved into the USSR. Shortly thereafter (in August 1941), the German euthanasia programme using gas came to an abrupt end (remaining Jewish candidates were sent east to the concentration camps). The reason is uncertain, though Müller-Hill suggests it may have been in order to free expertise and resources for the more pressing task of exterminating the Jewish populations of the conquered territories.[15] Certainly, equipment and personnel were sent east:

> So it was that doctors and other medical personnel in white coats supervised the process of exterminating Jews in the camps at Chelmno and Treblinka.[16] . . . From 9 March 1943, a licence to practise medicine was required of those making the 'selection' which took place on the railway ramps . . . and of those supervising the killing process in Auschwitz and other extermination camps . . . Auschwitz resembled the psychiatric institutions for extermination in that physicians were in charge of the 'selection' and killing. They had won these rights and were unwilling to have them taken away by others.[17]

In the light of this continuity with what followed, it is no surprise that the first victims of the orchestrated euthanasia programme were poisoned by carbon monoxide (and later cyanide) gas, naked, in extermination centres. Those selected for extermination included 'the mentally defective, psychotics (particularly schizophrenics), epileptics and patients suffering from infirmities of old age and from various organic neurologic disorders such as infantile paralysis, Parkinsonism, multiple sclerosis and brain tumors'. It was also here that the idea of disguising the gas chambers as showers originated. Alexander quotes Brack, '. . . who testified before Judge Sebring that the patients walked in calmly, deposited their towels and stood with their little pieces of soap under the shower outlets, waiting for the water to start running.' He adds: 'This statement was ample rebuttal of his claim that only the most severely regressed patients among the mentally sick and only the moribund ones among the physically sick were exterminated. In truth, all those unable to work and considered nonrehabilitable were killed.'[18]

A programme run on so substantial a scale could not be kept

hidden, and writers such as Proctor and Müller-Hill have demonstrated that it became widely known. There were many letters of protest, including some from public prosecutors and judges who found that those with whom they had a professional relationship had disappeared into one of the killing centres. Alexander offers an instance of a rare public protest, which itself illustrates the difficulty the authorities faced in keeping the programme from public view. A member of the Frankfurt-am-Main Court of Appeals wrote as follows:

> There is constant discussion of the question of the destruction of socially unfit life – in the places where there are mental institutions, in neighbouring towns, sometimes over a large area, throughout the Rhineland, for example. The people have come to recognize the vehicles in which the patients are taken from their original institution to the intermediate institution and from there to the liquidation institution. I am told that when they see these buses even the children call out: 'They're taking some more people to be gassed.' From Limburg it is reported that every day from one to three buses with shades drawn pass through on the way from Weilmunster to Hadamar, delivering inmates to the institution there. According to the stories the arrivals are immediately stripped to the skin, dressed in paper shirts, and forthwith taken to a gas chamber, where they are liquidated with hydrocyanic acid gas and an added anesthetic. The bodies are reported to be moved to a combustion chamber by means of a conveyor belt, six bodies to a furnace. The resulting ashes are then distributed into six urns which are shipped to the families. The heavy smoke from the crematory building is said to be visible over Hadamar every day. There is talk, furthermore, that in some cases heads and other portions of the body are removed for anatomical examination. The people working at this liquidation job in the institutions are said to be assigned from other areas and are shunned completely by the populace.[19]

There were other protests. 'Relatives, mental hospital administrators, and the Catholic and Protestant clergy of all ranks addressed questions and protests to the department of justice,' he writes. 'Among all the letters, I have not found one from a psychiatrist . . . ' Indeed, the full programme, which included electric shock therapy to encourage patients to return to work as well as euthanasia for those who could not, 'formed a package with which almost all German psychiatrists could fully identify.'[20]

No doubt because of such responses there was a continued awareness of the need to keep the programme as quiet as possible. It was obviously unpopular with the German public, and this reminds us of Freidson's observation that the medical profession is chiefly dependent not on public goodwill and support but on that of the ruling elite. The university-dominated medical profession, in which state patronage was wide and professional autonomy a charade, sought constantly to accommodate itself to the elite's requirements, and to march in step with the Nazi Party. A 1942 report recommends as follows:

> One of the essential requirements for carrying out euthanasia is that it should be as unobtrusive as possible . . . Orders for euthanasia must be given and executed entirely within the framework of the normal activity of the ward. Thus, with few exceptions, it should be difficult to distinguish euthanasia from a natural death . . . The fact that a few active psychiatrists with progressive attitudes have been practising medical euthanasia in their hospitals and that today a hospital can carry out medical euthanasia, even in a Catholic district, for long periods without attracting attention shows that this goal can be achieved.[21]

After the gassing programme, in which some 94,000 patients were killed, came to an end, a similar number died before the war ended from other causes – mainly brought on by cold, starvation and the forced work regimes.[22]

Further comment at this point is superfluous, save to quote Alexander's reflection on the relationship between the origins of the medical crimes and the awful end of the story:

> Whatever proportions these crimes finally assumed, it became evident to all who investigated them that they had started from small beginnings. The beginnings at first were merely a subtle shift in emphasis in the basic attitude of the physicians. It started with the acceptance of the attitude, basic to the euthanasia movement, that there is such a thing as life not worthy to be lived. This attitude in its early stages concerned itself merely

with the severely and chronic sick. Gradually the sphere of those to be included in this category was enlarged to encompass the socially unproductive, the ideologically unwanted, the racially unwanted and finally all non-Germans. But it is important to realize that the infinitely small wedged-in lever from which this entire trend of mind received its impetus was the attitude toward the nonrehabilitable sick.[23]

We have noted that the formal euthanasia programme (with its gassing centres) came to an end in August 1941. Public discontent may have been a contributory factor. Certainly, euthanasia continued to be practised – but in individual institutions, at the discretion of medical and administrative staffs. One contemporary account illustrates how this practice actually continued some months after the war had ended.[24]

Meanwhile, as Proctor states in *Racial Hygiene*:

Gas chambers at psychiatric institutions in southern and eastern Germany were dismantled and shipped east, where they were reinstalled at Belsen, Majdanek, Auschwitz, Treblinka, and Sobibor. The same doctors and technicians and nurses often followed the equipment. Germany's psychiatric hospitals forged the most important practical link between the destruction of the mentally ill and handicapped and the murder of Germany's ethnic and social minorities.[25]

THE MEDICAL EXPERIMENTS

As we have suggested, both in history and in ethics the euthanasia programme forms the context within which the programme of human experimentation was born. We could say more. There is little doubt that the programme played its part in paving the way to the Holocaust itself, and we have noted the role of the medical profession in administering the extermination programme. Yet too much must not be made of these connections. It is inevitable that we should trace the causes of both in the German intellectual environment of the preceding decades. Certainly, the medical profession itself (influenced, as we have seen, by psychiatrists above all) was prepared for its part in the developments of the war years by the experience of the euthanasia programme. Although doctors played many parts in the process of Holocaust, it is here in the area of experimental medical science that their role *as doctors* was plainest and most depraved.[26]

The political context must first be understood, since it was this which made human beings available to be employed as the subjects of deleterious experimentation. It was that same context in which slave labour was developed on a massive scale, and in which, of course, systematic extermination was the final feature.

Richard L. Rubenstein sums up the situation as follows:

> For the first time in history, a ruling elite in the heart of Europe, the center of Western civilization, had an almost inexhaustible supply of men and women with whom they could do anything they pleased, irrespective of any antique religious or moral prejudice. The Nazis had created a society of total domination. Among the preconditions for such a society are: (a) a bureaucratic administration capable of governing with utter indifference to the human needs of the inmates; (b) a supply of inmates capable of continuous replenishment; (c) the imposition of the death sentence on every inmate as soon as he or she enters.

In this situation, slave labour could be worked to death at whatever rate was determined to be most to the economic advantage of the state; and those within the system were at the disposal of any members of the elite who wished to make use of them. Rubenstein concludes: 'The Germans were able to create a society of total domination because of the competence of their police and civil service bureaucracies and because they possessed millions of totally superfluous men whose lives and sufferings were of absolutely no consequence to any power secular or sacred and who were as good as dead from the moment they entered the camps.'[27]

So Rubenstein goes on to speak of Auschwitz as 'the most thoroughgoing society of total domination in human history', since with the double purpose of the camp as a killing centre and a place of slave labour there was a class of slaves produced who 'could successfully be dealt with as things rather than human beings'. It had none of the ambiguity inherent in other slave systems, whether in antiquity or the *ante-bellum* South where, although slaves were deemed to be chattels, their treatment was by analogy with the treatment accorded to those who were citizens. Because from their entry into the camp the prisoners were already 'doomed', set apart for death, theirs could be the ultimately degrading treatment.[28]

As a result, 'In a society of total domination, there is absolutely no moral limit on the uses normal, perverse, or obscene to which the masters can put the human beings at their disposal.' A prime use which emerged for those thus totally dominated, and entirely devoid of rights in law or in sentiment, was that of human guinea pigs in the hands of ever-energetic medical–scientific research. 'Once German physicians realized that they had an almost limitless supply of human beings at their disposal for experiments, some very respectable professors at medical schools and research institutes seized the unique opportunity.'[29]

And it was, from their point of view, a very good opportunity indeed. The employment of apes and dogs as surrogates for humans in all manner of experimentation was so plainly superseded by the possibility of using the real thing that it is almost strange that, once the principle had been accepted, more use was not made of the 'material' afforded by the camps. Of course, the explanation lies in the situation of war; it is no surprise that many of the experimental programmes which found this material of special use were those concerned, directly or indirectly, with the prosecution of the war. Had Nazi Germany not been defeated, its post-war science would have had continued access to a pool of human research subjects who had no legal standing. It is not hard to speculate on the kind of uses to which they would have been put.

One of the connections which may be traced between the euthanasia programme and the camp experiments lies in the experimental use of brain and other tissues from euthanasia victims. There was much interest in the sudden availability of human brains, and one researcher wrote in 1944 of having received a total of 697. He published one 'interesting' piece of research on the brain of a child whose mother had been gassed (with carbon monoxide) during pregnancy. Its most interesting feature was its date of publication – 1949 – when he was continuing to work on 'material' gathered during the war. The collection still exists.[30]

Another area of research, this time on living human beings, was concerned with the racial purity programme and aimed to develop an effective and cheap process of mass sterilisation – for use on various groups, especially Jews who had married Christians and been baptised. What better way than to devise various possible methods, and then test them? One set of experiments was carried out in a special block built at Auschwitz, under the direction of Professor Clausberg. He sought to induce sterilisation by means of intra-uterine injections of various substances. The process was extremely painful, and some women actually died as a result. The (unrealised) hope was to produce 1,000 sterilisations a day.[31]

Viktor Brack, a civil servant, proposed another method to Himmler, this time in the context of concern to sterilise some 3 million of the 10 million Jews so they could be kept alive as slave labour. X-ray machines would be built into desks at which groups of 100 men were to be asked to complete forms while they were unwittingly sterilised. In the event, when this was tried on some hundreds of men in Auschwitz it failed because the men were severely burned.[32]

A further category of experiments was also connected with the conduct of the war, although it covered a wide variety of perceived needs on the part of the state. One was that of an effective and undetectable means of killing troublesome individuals, whether high-ranking Nazis who had fallen foul of their superiors, or particular prisoners whose death might lead to embarrassment if foul play were suspected. Several methods were tried. One involved the artificial stimulation of septicaemia, and trials were run in several camps. At Dachau, Alexander notes, 'the subjects were almost exclusively Polish Catholic priests'. Yet it did not prove wholly successful.

Another method involved 'repeated intravenous injections of live tubercle bacilli, which brought on acute miliary tuberculosis within a few weeks'. So that even SS colleagues could not guess what purpose this work might serve, the preliminary tests 'were performed exclusively on children'.

Clearly, any such selective method of murder would involve a physician. In the altogether more mundane context of life on a German U-boat, it was he who was charged with the elimination of trouble-makers by lethal injection. 'Whatever methods he used,' Alexander continues, 'the physician gradually became the unofficial executioner, for the sake of convenience, informality and relative secrecy.'[33]

A series of experiments was conducted in Dachau in support of the strictly military concerns of the German state by Dr Sigmund Rascher. Himmler sought a blood coagulant to help stem battlefield haemorrhage, and once it was developed Rascher tested it by counting and timing drops of blood from the freshly-cut stumps of conscious amputees. Concern for the effects of decompression at high altitude led to tests on subjects in a mobile decompression chamber. Severe symptoms were noted: 'Convulsions, then unconsciousness in which the body was hanging limp and later, after wakening, temporary blindness, paralysis or severe confusional twilight states.' Rascher sought the cause, and 'placed the subjects of the experiment under water and dissected them while the heart was still beating, demonstrating air embolism in the blood vessels of the heart, liver, chest wall and brain.' A third series of experiments concerned the effects of exposure to cold (arising from the experience of airmen who ditched in the sea). Rascher used some 300 Dachau prisoners in these tests, of whom eighty to ninety died. 'In one report on this work Rascher asked permission to shift these experiments from Dachau to Auschwitz, a larger camp where they might cause less disturbance because the subjects shrieked from pain when their extremities froze white.' It took six or seven hours in ice-cold water to kill a man wearing airman's kit.[34]

Finally, there were experiments which were unconnected with the needs of the war, opportunistic exercises in research. The most famous concerned twins, and especially gypsy twins, whom Josef Mengele selected on disembarkation from the trains which brought new inmates to Auschwitz, at the same time as the selection was made of those who would shortly be gassed (chiefly women, children and the elderly) and those destined for slave labour. He collected over 100 pairs of twins, together with a similar number of families of dwarfs and deformed persons. A range of tests and experiments was conducted, including the infecting of pairs of twins with typhoid bacteria to observe whether the disease ran the same course in each. In another report we read that Mengele had four pairs of twins killed by intracardiac injection so that their eye peculiarities could be studied.[35]

A final example of opportunistic research may be offered, though here the motivation was different:

> One of the most revolting experiments was the testing of sulfonamides against gas gangrene by Professor Gebhardt and his collaborators, for which young women captured from the Polish Resistance Movement served as subjects. Necrosis was produced in a muscle of the leg by ligation and the wound was infected with various types of gas-gangrene bacilli; frequently, dirt, pieces of wood and glass splinters were added to the wound. Some of these victims died, and others sustained severe mutilating deformities of the leg.[36]

And why? 'Dr Gebhardt performed these experiments to clear himself of the suspicion that he had contributed to the death of SS General Reinhard ('The Hangman') Heydrich, either negligently or deliberately, by failing to treat his wound infection with sulfonamides,' after the (ultimately successful) attempt on Heydrich's life.[37]

THE RECONSTRUCTION OF HIPPOCRATISM?

We have noted that the best evidence of the degree to which German medicine was involved in these events *as medicine*, and not merely by implication in the cause of total war, is the response they elicited from the post-war international medical community. In the face of such a wholesale departure from the Hippocratic tradition by a nation in the heart of European Christendom, it was felt necessary to re-state the Hippocratic values.

Yet, as we shall see, in their very re-statement these values underwent subtle change. Their re-statement proved to be a re-structuring, in conscious contradistinction to Nazi medicine yet at the same time in unconscious deviation from Hippocratism proper.

The judgment which closed the medical trials at Nuremberg included a statement of medical ethical principles which has become known as the Nuremberg Code. The Code sets out basic criteria for experiments involving human subjects, and it has been the basis for later declarations with similar intent. Twenty-three defendants, mostly doctors, had appeared on charges arising out of experiments on human subjects, and the Code sought to clarify the principles which had been assumed by the International Military Tribunal in the trial of these cases. The Code consists of ten statements of principle, the first and most important of which is that those who participate in such experiments must freely consent. Others cover the value of the results which the work is expected to yield and the need for the experiments themselves to be conducted safely.[38]

Wilkinson comments on the 'great historical importance' of the Code, by which he intends to refer to its path-finding significance for later ethical statements. Yet it is also of historical significance as the representative response of the international community to what had taken place. Wilkinson observes that though the Code originated in a judicial context, its force is ethical. 'It cannot, therefore, constitute a safeguard against the kind of criminal behaviour allowed under the Nazi regime. Such a safeguard can only be found in the presuppositions, character and integrity of the experimenter.' The meaning of this statement is not entirely clear, since if everything depends on the character of the experimenter there is no 'safeguard' at all, just a hope that experimenters will be good men and women. What the Code crucially lacks are two basic elements which are characteristic of the Hippocratic Oath, and we return to them shortly; they are absent also from other contemporary attempts at the re-construction of Hippocratism.

The most important of these attempts at re-stating the tradition followed on the heels of the Nuremberg Code. In that same year, 1948, the World Medical Association was founded. In the next year its Assembly met in Geneva and approved what was intended to be a self-conscious re-writing of the Hippocratic Oath, re-affirming Hippocratism in the face of the shame and tragedy of the German medical experience. It is worth quoting this summary statement of post-war medical ethics, the Declaration of Geneva, as it sought to re-pristinate Hippocratism.

> I solemnly pledge myself to consecrate my life to the service of humanity;
> I will give to my teachers the respect and gratitude which is their due;
> I will practise my profession with conscience and dignity;

The health of my patient will be my first consideration;

I will respect the secrets which are confided in me;

I will maintain by all the means in my power, the honour and the noble traditions of the medical profession;

My colleagues will be my brothers;

I will not permit considerations of religion, nationality, race, party politics or social standing to intervene between my duty and my patient;

I will maintain the utmost respect for human life from the time of conception; even under threat. I will not use my medical knowledge contrary to the laws of humanity;

I make these promises solemnly, freely and upon my honour.[39]

While the Declaration deliberately echoes the phrasing of the Hippocratic Oath, it is a very different kind of document. For one thing, it is entirely secular. The character of the Oath is necessarily religious, and whether set in the context of ancient Pythagorean paganism or re-interpreted within the Christian tradition, it is an oath, sworn in the presence of the physician's God; an ethical statement deriving its force from its context in theism.

By comparison, the Declaration is a pallid affirmation made by the physician in the presence of man alone. For all its self-proclaimed solemnity, its only points of reference are horizontal. The act of displacing an oath with a declaration bears powerful witness to the secularising of the western medical tradition. Even in 1948, as medicine sought to gird up its loins in post-war reconstruction, all it could look to was itself: 'the honour and noble traditions of the medical profession'. No longer did it understand itself as answerable to God, nor recognise that it was in its transcendent character that the 'honour and noble traditions' of medicine had their origin and their moral force.

So, far from the ringing re-assertion of Hippocratism which it is alleged to be (and which its framers no doubt intended), the Declaration reads as a lament to a lost medical tradition. The physicians of the Reich did not destroy that tradition, though what they did makes sense only as the medicine of those already living in its twilight, who forged their way ruthlessly ahead into darkness. The World Medical Association, in attempting the re-institution of the tradition, discovered that its life-blood had run out. Its values, more or less, remained; but they had all the substance of the smile of the Cheshire cat. The vertical dimension, which provided not only formal sanction but the material dynamic of Hippocratism, had gone. The religious–philosophical imperatives of the Pythagorean–Judaeo–Christian tradition could no longer command the loyalty of the international medical community. The party was over.

We have called this dimension 'vertical', but it is perhaps better to speak of it as transcendental. Hippocratism was from start to finish a transcendental medical faith, forever reaching beyond itself for its ontological ground and self-understanding. Its ethical injunctions – its code, as it were – were inseparable from its covenantal structure and the self-involving character of the physician's calling. In taking up the medical task he committed himself to his God, to his patient, and to his profession (to his teacher). These were no contingent, optional commitments. They were of the essence of his medicine, and it is for that reason that he can solemnly swear never to divulge his medical expertise to any who has not first taken this irrevocable existential step of moral commitment. The contrast with the two-dimensional and self-consciously secular ethics of post-theistic Geneva could hardly be greater; indeed, it is actually heightened by the implicit intention of the Declaration to stand in the Hippocratic line, and by its *de facto* ethical continuity. The Declaration of Geneva, drafted as 'a sort of updated version of the Hippocratic Oath'[40] and supposed by many to be a proud re-statement of that victorious tradition is – all unknowing – both a lament to a lost, transcendent tradition and a fanfare to post-Hippocratic medicine.

Its achievement was to clear the ground for the substantive ethical changes which would soon follow. The Hippocratic Oath, with its transcendental, covenantal structure, holds firmly together as an integrated whole. The Declaration of Geneva is a series of ethical assertions which invite amendment and revision. This judgment may seem harsh, for the goodwill of those who framed the Declaration was great and their loyalty to their tradition strong – as was their profound abhorrence of the German experience. Yet this is what happened.

The penultimate clause of the Declaration states: 'I will maintain the utmost respect for human life from the time of conception.' Already this is distinct from the Oath, since the Oath uses negatives – in order to ensure clarity and fixity in the ethical tradition, and the idea of 'respect for life' is malleable in a way in which the Hippocratic forswearing of abortion and suicide–euthanasia could never be. At the same time, the Declaration seeks in this phrase to echo the Oath. And it does so by implying the fundamental continuity of human life 'from the time of conception'. Though this is not how the Oath deals with the problem of abortion, we do know that this was the Pythagorean view.

Should we be surprised that this key ethical provision in the Declaration of Geneva has subsequently been modified? The whole matter can be confusing, for the Declaration is sometimes quoted as if the original wording of this clause had never been.[41] In fact, the 1960s amendment of the penultimate clause from 'utmost respect for human life from the time of conception' to 'utmost respect . . . from its beginning' is of high significance. As well as marking, by implication, the formal departure of the medical community from one of the key prescriptions of its tradition, this act of amendment leads us to fear for the standing of the Declaration and every other such statement of medical ethics. By abandoning the transcendent and covenantal character of the Oath, those who drafted this reformulation of Hippocratism have turned the principles of medical ethics into one long composite motion to be debated year on year at representative medical assemblies.

And the focal point of our critique of the Declaration lies just here, in the fact that it is the kind of statement which invites amendment. It has been followed by many other statements, all implicitly claiming to stand within the Hippocratic tradition, all at the same time distancing themselves from it and failing to capture its genius by their two-dimensional ethics and the static, formal character of their injunctions. Elsewhere we draw attention to the manner in which fundamental change takes place in a profession, and to the importance (to the profession) of accomplishing change while maintaining an appearance of faithfulness to the tradition. It is not proposed that the tradition be abandoned and a new one set in its place. Every shift in the tradition is justified by reference to the tradition and claimed as a clarification or up-dating of that tradition. Changes in form are the point of departure for changes in substance. There could be no better example than the Declaration of Geneva. Why did the World Medical Association not simply swear anew the Hippocratic Oath?

Notes

1   This development is chronicled in compelling detail in Robert Proctor, *Racial Hygiene: Medicine under the Nazis*, Harvard University Press, Cambridge, Mass., and London, 1988. The reason we summarise these developments here is two-fold: they represent the historical backcloth to the Nuremberg Code and Declaration of Geneva, which are the starting-points of contemporary medical ethics; and they illustrate drastically the implications of abandoning the human values at the heart of the humane medical tradition. As we see in the following chapter, the question of deleterious experimentation on human subjects re-emerges in post-war abuse of the fetus and embryo. However much we may deplore these practices, we do not suggest a connection, historical or ideological; and there is no doubt that most of those who have been involved in these practices believe in good faith that they are practising moral medicine. Yet that, of course, is part of the problem, and not the least part.

2   *Ibid.*, p. 178.

3   Benno Müller-Hill, *Murderous Science*, Oxford University Press, 1988, p. 11.

4   *Ibid.*, pp. 12f.

5   Proctor, *Racial Hygiene*, p. 193.

6   *Ibid.*, p. 191.

7   *Ibid.*, p. 192.

8   Müller-Hill, *Murderous Science*, pp. 102f, and Proctor, *Racial Hygiene*, p. 280.

9   *Ibid.*, p. 38.

10 Leo Alexander, 'Medical Science under Dictatorship', *New England Journal of Medicine* 241:2 (1949), repr. in *Ethics and Medicine* 3:3 (1987) and in *Death without Dignity: Euthanasia in Perspective*, edited by the present writer, Rutherford House, Edinburgh, 1990.

11 Alexander, p. 40.

12 *Ibid.*
13 Müller-Hill, *Murderous Science*, pp. 40f; Alexander, 'Medical Science under Dictatorship', p. 40.
14 Müller-Hill, *Murderous Science*, p. 41; cp. Proctor, *Racial Hygiene*, pp. 189f.
15 Müller-Hill, *Murderous Science*, pp. 41, 46.
16 *Ibid.*, p. 48.
17 *Ibid.*, p. 55.
18 Alexander, 'Medical Science under Dictatorship', p. 40.
19 *Ibid.*, p. 40. He adds laconically: 'Here one sees what "euthanasia" means in actual practice.'
20 Müller-Hill, *Murderous Science*, p. 43.
21 Cited in *ibid.*, p. 64.
22 *Ibid.*, p. 64.
23 Alexander, 'Medical Science under Dictatorship', p. 44.
24 Proctor, *Racial Hygiene*, p. 192. Three months after the occupation of Germany it took a detachment of US soldiers to stop the routine killing of mental patients in one hospital.
25 *Ibid.*, p. 212.
26 One of the most important sources for the details which follow is A. Mitscherlich and F. Mielke, *Doctors of Infamy: the Story of the Nazi Medical Crimes*, first published in English (in New York) in 1949 from the German original of 1947 published by Henry Schuman. Subsequent editions have used more than one title.
27 Richard L. Rubenstein, *The Cunning of History*, Harper & Row, New York, 1975, pp. 34f.
28 *Ibid.*, pp. 46f.
29 *Ibid.*, pp. 48f.
30 Müller-Hill, *Murderous Science*, pp. 66f.
31 Rubenstein, *The Cunning of History*, pp. 50f; Alexander, 'Medical Science under Dictatorship', p. 41.
32 Rubenstein, *The Cunning of History*, p. 51; Alexander, 'Medical Science under Dictatorship', p. 41, who adds: 'I myself examined 4 castrated survivors of this ghastly experiment. Three had extensive necrosis of the skin near the genitalia, and the other an extensive necrosis of the urethra.'
33 Alexander, 'Medical Science under Dictatorship', p. 42.
34 *Ibid.*, pp. 42f.
35 Müller-Hill, *Murderous Science*, pp. 71f.
36 Alexander, 'Medical Science under Dictatorship', pp. 43f.

37 *Ibid.*, p. 44.
38 The Code is reproduced in various places, most recently in J. Wilkinson, *Christian Ethics in Health Care*, pp. 346f.
39 This version is given in A. V. Campbell, *Moral Dilemmas in Medicine*, Second Edition, Churchill Livingston, Edinburgh and New York, 1975, p. 197. A revised version is now current, and is available in John Wilkinson, *Christian Ethics in Health Care*, Handsel Press, Edinburgh, 1988, p. 149; in which, in addition to small changes in punctuation, the penultimate clause reads (without comment) 'respect for human life *from its beginning*' in place of 'from conception' (our emphasis). See *The Handbook of Medical Ethics*, British Medical Association, London, 1984.
40 Ranaan Gillon, *Philosophical Medical Ethics*, John Wiley, Chichester, 1986, p. 9. The assumption of the essential continuity between the Oath and post-Hippocratic 'oaths' is well-nigh universal. So the *Oxford Reference Dictionary* informs us that the Hippocratic Oath 'is still taken, in various modified forms, by those who qualify as medical practitioners'.
41 As in Wilkinson, *Christian Ethics in Health Care*, for example.

4

The Margins of the Human Race

In the opening chapters we devoted much space to the question of the character of the Hippocratic tradition, the nature of Hippocratism. But what is the key to our understanding of contemporary *post*-Hippocratic medicine? Let us attempt a candid analysis. Its most characteristic feature is the progressive marginalisation of those who are weakest and most powerless in the clinical situation. This analysis is not only candid – it will be considered by some to be highly provocative. Who will admit to medicine as an exercise of power over the powerless? That would imply a vicious parody of Hippocratic paternalism, in an emergent post-Hippocratism in which patient autonomy has become a watchword. Yet is it simply absurd? We argue in this chapter and the one following that such a picture of recent developments and current trends offers us a coherent pattern of understanding and interpretation.

Needless to say, the manner in which this has come about is complex. It has been partly unconscious, reflecting changes in values in the society in which medicine is practised. We have noted that it is in the nature of a profession that changes in professional values come about slowly and imperceptibly, unacknowledged and unrecognised, save by the few. This is the only way in which fundamental change *can* take place in an institution which is held together by its consciousness of the tradition of which it is guardian. The displacement of the Hippocratic ethic of philanthropic service by a new ethic of power has, unsurprisingly, gone unacknowledged. Since it represents a betrayal not only of Hippocratism but of values widely claimed in contemporary society, its potent significance remains largely hidden. And, of course, much actual medical practice continues according to patterns long-established. It is in the nature of the case that change comes about imperceptibly; and that, in many situations, the old medicine and the new nearly or entirely overlap in their prescription for patient care. Yet something very fundamental has changed; though the passengers may remain unaware, the ship's course has been altered.

Yet if post-Hippocratism is a medicine of power, of whose power over whom? It is not that the post-Hippocratic doctor exercises some kind of personal power over his patient to his own gain (though in some cases this may be so). More typically, he is an agent of someone else, whose opportunity for power over his patient is the by-product of the clinical situation. This may take the form of the power of one individual over another, of the community as a whole over some of its members, or of one class within the community over another class. The key role played by medicine is that of an agency acting on behalf of another. The physician is the representative of the community and, just as he represents the community in caring for the sick, so he does when the community wishes to care for them no longer (and, indeed, in 'not caring' also for those who are *not* sick, but who for some other reason are within his power). He works in the name and the power, therefore, of those who give him authority to act. On their behalf he may become the midwife not of life but of death.

Over whom does he exercise power, on their behalf? Over the weak and powerless, those members of the human community who are disadvantaged in such a manner that the community itself has come to regard their membership of the community as ambiguous and open to question.

The next section of this chapter offers an inventory of those who find themselves in this position today. How has the contemporary medical profession, which takes its point of departure in the Declaration of Geneva, so regarded them as to place them outside of its canons, or to interpret those canons in such a way as to provide for their special treatment? The image which we suggest best fits this process is offered in the title of this chapter. We see in our generation a progressive marginalisation of certain classes of the human race. They are already on the margins of social standing and influence. The margins to which they are being pressed are the margins of human dignity and, accordingly, of human rights; the margins of the right to be treated as human beings at all.

We suggest this model partly because it covers two different groups of human beings. Some are widely considered to be beyond the margins of humanity. The best example is that of the early human embryo, the candidate for deleterious and destructive experimentation. In other cases, by contrast, there is little denying that those whose treatment is under consideration are fellow human beings. Perhaps the best example here is that of the handicapped newborn, the candidates now for euthanasia. As we see later, some writers in medical ethics debate what it means to be human, or what it is about being human that makes humans, or some humans, morally significant – 'morally relevant characteristics', to use Peter Singer's phrase. Yet, as discussion goes forward, this is of decreasing interest. Having taken leave of Hippocratism, in which even abortion and the aiding in suicide of those wishing to die are forbidden, we have arrived at a position in which whole classes of human beings have their humanity declared at best ambiguous. They are outside, or perhaps just inside, the margins of the human race.

Putative definitions of humanity are now legion. So it is no surprise that in one of the most significant documents of our time, the 1984 Warnock Report (the work of a committee set up by the British government to address the problems raised by the new reproductive technology), there is a deliberate avoidance of the question of 'whether' the early embryo is to be regarded as human 'or not' – in favour of the practical issue of 'how it is right to treat' the embryo. By ducking the central issue in the debate, they merely illustrate the increasing irrelevance of that issue in contemporary discussion. Interest is focused in the practical question: how is it right to treat this case? The ambiguous humanity of those who have been consigned to the borders of the human race does not offer the guidance that is sought. The question of whether they are just inside or just outside those borders is seen to be as irrelevant to the practical conclusions as it is, perhaps, unanswerable on the premises of those who ask it. Though they have a lingering suspicion that it must mean something, they are no longer sure what it means to be human; so 'whether or not' it is human has ceased to matter. Since, to those outside the narrow confines of bioethical discussion, this suspicion remains so strong that it means everything though they are not sure why, those within feel obliged to address it. But the two-dimensional character of post-war ethics has given room to manoeuvre out of the orbit of Hippocratism altogether. The early embryo, as plainly, wholly human as it is plainly, wholly powerless, is the index of life on the margins of the race.

A TAXONOMY OF THE POWERLESS

By focusing on the idea of patient powerlessness and on medicine as an occasion for the abuse of power, we draw attention to assumptions that lie behind the relationship of patient and physician and, in turn, behind the way both doctors and society view human nature and human value.

We turn first to discuss particular cases before returning in the next chapter to the general considerations which we have outlined. One of the principal issues underlying this debate is how an over-riding concern with the relief of suffering is undermining the sanctity of life. It is to this theme that we turn in the next chapter.

The Ancient Context of Contemporary Debate

One of the major handicaps of public (and much professional) discussion is the isolation of contemporary life-and-death concerns from their history. This ignorance has largely served the cause of those who have sought change in the Hippocratic consensus. The notion that fundamental ethical challenges are posed by specifically modern circumstances (such as improvements in medical technique) leads to a disorientation and impoverishment of understanding. We lose the historical and ethical perspective provided by the recognition that these questions are ancient as well as modern. The impression is sometimes given that the new ethics are simply a spin-off of the new technology. Nothing could be further from the truth.

Of course, it is true both that the new ethical options are on offer for the first time in many centuries, and that they are on offer in a climate of unprecedented technical advance. In every area of medical technique – drug therapy, surgical skills, the application of the new electronics – medicine is brimming over with extraordinary developments. They certainly pose their own ethical problems, not least in the area of resource allocation. But the issues of life and death which form the boundaries of the medical enterprise remain unchanged, though focused afresh in every new context of technique. So ultrasonography has revolutionised ante-natal care and, in the process, offered new diagnostic techniques for fetal abnormality.[1] Yet we cannot discuss the ethics of abortion for fetal handicap apart from its double context in the ancient debate about abortion and the equally ancient practice of infanticide of the handicapped.

We have already considered the significance of the Hippocratic Oath in the medicine of Greek antiquity. As Edelstein has shown, in its distinct ethical injunctions it sets the Hippocratic physician against prevailing trends in medical and general social practice. The inference which some interpreters have drawn, that this observation relativises and effectively discounts the importance of the Hippocratic tradition, needs to be assessed in the context of what we know about those medical and general social practices to which the Hippocratic physicians took exception. Since the critics of Hippocratism seek to set aside its life-and-death ethical matrix embodied in ancient opposition to abortion and suicide–euthanasia, their desire is evidently for a renewal of the pre-Hippocratic medical and social values. We return to this theme later. First we sketch some further details of the practices against which the Pythagorean physicians protested in their manifesto.

Their concern was precisely for those whom we have identified as powerless in the clinical situation. Indeed, that is how a writer in the major work of reference, Hastings' *Encyclopaedia of Religion and Ethics*, approaches the question in its ancient context. 'The most helpless of mankind are those who have just begun life, and those who, through old age or infirmity, are about to leave it.'[2] We find this comment in the context of a discussion of exposure (of infants) and abandonment (of aged or infirm adults). It is dangerous to generalise about attitudes in Greek antiquity, since there was a pluriformity of approach to these as to other questions. Yet there is no disagreement that the Hippocratic ethics (according to Edelstein the medical application of the Pythagoreanism of the later fourth century BC) stand in marked contrast to the prevailing attitudes in Greek society, which were reflected in its mainstream medical traditions. As we have seen, Edelstein's judgment is clear: 'Suicide was not censured in antiquity. Abortion was practised in Greek times no less than in the Roman era, and it was resorted to without scruple. Small wonder! In a world in which it was held justifiable to expose children immediately after birth, it would hardly seem objectionable to destroy the embryo.'[3] And in these three sentences Edelstein sums up the three areas in which Greek antiquity regarded human life as disposable: before birth, immediately after birth, and when through age or infirmity it became a burden.

To begin with the last, Edelstein summarises the position as follows:

> Platonists, Cynics and Stoics . . . held suicide permissible for the diseased. Some of these philosophers even extolled such an act as the greatest triumph of men over fate. Aristotle, on the other hand, claimed that it was cowardly to give in to bodily pain, and Epicurus admonished men not to be subdued by illness . . . [Yet] the Aristotelian and Epicurean opposition to suicide did not involve moral censure. If men decided to take their lives, they were within their rights as sovereign masters of themselves. The Aristotelian and Epicurean schools condoned suicide . . . Pythagoreanism, then, remains the only philosophical dogma that can possibly account for the attitude advocated in the Hippocratic Oath. For indeed among all Greek thinkers the Pythagoreans alone outlawed suicide and did so without qualification.[4]

The reason was theological. Suicide was an affront to God, since (in the Pythagorean view) 'the soul is undergoing in the body a penitential discipline for ante-natal sin. Hence suicide is an unwarranted rebellion against the will of God on the part of the individual, whom it behoves to wait until it please God to set him free.'[5]

If the practice of medical suicide in ancient Greece offers us an example which may be set alongside voluntary euthanasia in contemporary debate, the widespread practice of abandonment (the exposure to death of the elderly and infirm) offers us a parallel to euthanasia that is involuntary. This was not common in ancient Greece, though it did happen. Strabo records the 'law of Ceos', which prevented 'him who was unable to live well from living ill'.[6] In many primitive societies, ancient and modern, the elderly and infirm have been abandoned to the forces of nature, and in some cases deliberately killed.

We turn next to the analogous practice of the exposure of infants. Unlike the abandonment of the elderly and infirm, this is known to have been common in ancient Greece, as in other societies. The *Encyclopaedia of Religion and Ethics* defines it in these terms: 'When [the] neglect of children takes the form of removing them from the mother's habitation and leaving them unprotected to perish by starvation, the elements, or wild beasts, or to be rescued by the chance passer-by, it is called *Exposure*.'[7]

In the *Encyclopaedia* the writer continues with a survey of this practice among primitive peoples in his day – the opening years of the twentieth century:

> . . . exposure is often only one of many methods of infanticide. The populations among which it is most common are those which live by hunting or as nomad herdsmen. Thus, amongst the native tribes of South-East Australia it is usual to kill infants by starvation, first by depriving them of food in the camp, and, when they become peevish, removing them to a distance and leaving them to die . . . In the South Sea Islands the same end is achieved by drowning or burying alive . . . The Koniagas, a tribe of Eskimos, abandon girls in the wilderness after stuffing grass into their mouths . . . Amongst the Arabs before Muhammad the same system prevailed, and is referred to frequently in the Qur'an as a practice to be forbidden. Here sons were preserved, but daughters were usually buried alive.[8]

The early influence of Islam is noteworthy in the light of our comments in Chapter One on the influence of Hippocratism in mediaeval Arab medicine.

We turn now to the practice in classical antiquity. Jones writes as follows of what he regards as a product of 'luxury and selfishness':

> In many countries . . . an improvement in the standard of living is accompanied by a disinclination to rear children. From the 4th cent. B.C. onwards, this was conspicuous in Greece, and in Rome it formed a theme of discussion for philosophers and satirists. How common the practice of exposure was, may be gathered from the frequency with which the heroines of the New Comedy, who come before us in the Latin versions of Plautus and Terence, are represented as having been exposed.[9]

Plato himself advocated the exposure of all sickly children.[10]

It is interesting to note that the reason exposure was practised in Greece, rather than other forms of infanticide, lay in the conviction that, even if it resulted in death (which sometimes, perhaps often, it did not; since the childless, or those for whom a child was of some economic value, would rescue the child), it was regarded as guilt-free. 'So long as a man did not kill the infant with his own hands, he had no serious scruples about leaving it to perish of starvation.' The parallels in contemporary discussion are striking.[11]

The practice of abortion was also widespread among primitive peoples, as it was in classical antiquity, although one authoritative survey can state: 'Destruction of the human embryo [taken here to include the fetus] has not among any people become a social habit, as general infanticide has done among some modern primitive communities and among the ancient Greeks and Italians.'[12]

No doubt one reason was the risk to the mother, which could be high – higher than that of childbirth (which could be followed by exposure). Risks notwithstanding, abortion has been widespread among primitive as among civilised peoples, and it was a commonplace of the Graeco–Roman world. Another scholar writes as follows:

> From the earliest days of ancient Greece and Rome to the time of Augustine, abortion was practised frequently by pagans and

occasionally by Jews and Christians. It seems to have been more common among the wealthy than among the poor: Juvenal wrote of how seldom a 'gilded bed' contained a pregnant woman because abortion was so readily available to the rich. But the poor aborted too, as did married and unmarried, chaste and prostitute. Other people beside pregnant women were involved in abortion. A husband or lover might force a woman to abort. Certain doctors performed nontherapeutic as well as therapeutic abortions. Amateur and paid abortionists and dealers in abortifacient drugs were available.[13]

And if we may cite Edelstein once more:

Most of the Greek philosophers even commended abortion. For Plato, foeticide is one of the regular institutions of the ideal state. Whenever the parents are beyond that age which he thinks best for the begetting of children, the embryo should be destroyed. Aristotle reckons abortion the best procedure to keep the population within the limits which he considers essential for a well-ordered community . . .

To be sure, one limitation apparently is recognised by ancient philosophers. Aristotle advocates that abortion should be performed before the foetus has attained animal life; after that time he no longer considers abortion compatible with holiness. But such a restriction is based on the biological notion that the embryo from a certain time on partakes in animal life. Other philosophers and scientists, in fact most of them, including the Platonists and the Stoics, denied that such was the case. Animation, they thought, began at the moment of birth. Therefore, in their opinion, abortion must have been permissible throughout pregnancy.

However, with the Pythagoreans it was different:

They held that the embryo was an animate being from the moment of conception . . . Consequently, for the Pythagoreans, abortion, whenever practised, meant destruction of a living being. Granted that the righteousness of abortion depends on whether the embryo is animate or not, the Pythagoreans could not but reject abortion unconditionally.[14]

What is particularly interesting here is Edelstein's explanation of the logic of the Pythagorean position. In harmony with others in ancient Greece, the Pythagoreans opposed the taking of life after animation had been held to occur. Yet for them the point of animation lay at the beginning. There was no such thing as an 'inanimate' embryo or fetus, so there could be no ethical abortion. Once more, the parallels in contemporary society are striking.

Feticide and Fetal Abuse

The profoundly ambiguous character of fetal life in the law and medicine of the West is partly a reflection of the ambiguity of the gestational state itself. But it is, of course, something more. It reflects essentially post-Christian uncertainty about human nature, an uncertainty which has given rise to widespread discussion of the single principle which seemed for so long non-negotiable, the principle of the sanctity of human life. So James Rachels, in his recent defence of euthanasia entitled *The End of Life*, is able to be candid as few defenders of euthanasia have been before: 'Where killing is concerned,' he says, 'I believe that the dominant moral tradition of our culture is, in fact, contrary to reason.'[15]

Our uncertainty as to what it means to be human is leading to the denial that 'being human' itself carries any special moral significance. So those at the margins of human existence – the young, the old, the sick – begin to partake of an ambiguity essentially analogous with that of the fetus. One fruit of this trend in bioethical thinking, in relativising the significance of human being itself, is to render increasingly uninteresting the answer to the question 'When does life begin?', which seemed once to be a, if not the, major question in bioethical discussion. For once the intrinsic 'sanctity', which in our ethical tradition attached to every human life, is withdrawn, the question whether, at a given stage, embryonic or fetal life is to be considered 'human life' like ours, begins to fade in significance. Much more pressing is the need for an *ad hoc* judgment about the worth which we seek to confer on a particular human life, whether young or old, *in vitro* or *in vivo*.

There is a growing tendency to abandon the central conviction of our medical tradition, itself inter-related with the basis of our concepts of human rights, that there is such a thing as 'human life' with a dignity which is intrinsic and, therefore, with an inalienable moral standing. If there is not, then discussion concerning at what stage, or through which particular developmental process, the gestational human child takes on a particular character is an exercise in futility. Human dignity and worth are not recognised as inhering in (all) human being, they are conferred on (some) human being – that which conforms with a given set of criteria.

The ethical debate which used to centre on the question of abortion now has twin *foci* in the traditional fetus/abortion issue and the new issue of the embryo and the possibility of its use in deleterious research. Embryo research has undoubtedly set the question of the status of pre-natal human life in a new and sharper perspective. The development of *in vitro* fertilisation (IVF) has turned the question of the use and abuse of the early embryo, so recently hypothetical, into one of the great public policy issues of the day.

Yet, at the same time, these two sets of questions lie at the centre of two generally separate discussions. The abortion debate has broken its conventional moorings in the 'When does life begin?' discussion, and moved toward a broader analogy with the issues of life and death *ex utero* (to which we turn later). Support for the infanticide of handicapped newborns, and classic discussions of euthanasia now rooted in widespread (formal and informal) practice, have helped construct a new framework in which induced abortion is frankly understood as an act of ante-natal euthanasia.

A striking example is to be found in a recent magazine article written by a mother who had consented to abortion after the diagnosis of Down's Syndrome. After telling the story of her pregnancy and the shock the diagnosis caused, she writes of her mixed emotions:

> Of course, when I went to bed I couldn't sleep. I know it sounds awful, but I hated the baby because it wasn't right and it kicked all night as if somehow it felt the hatred. Next morning I felt better and realised that although this baby wasn't going to go full term, it was still my baby. The hate suddenly turned into overwhelming love . . . We knew we'd be invited to see our baby, our Wreford. I knew it was a boy. I just knew. We'd agreed on names . . . a girl would be Sarah after my mother, a boy Wreford, after Bob's dad. This was Wreford . . .
>
> At last it was over. Wreford was born. He was quickly taken away and then so gently, this young doctor invited us to look

at him. He pointed out the already enlarged tongue and other tell-tale features. But although we could see these, Wreford was really so beautiful that I just couldn't cry . . .

I think about Wreford often. He was born the day after my mother's birthday and I'm glad he wasn't born earlier because now he's got his own day and I can set that aside for him – to think about how much he has meant to me and look at the photo of him the hospital gave me.

Despite the trauma and the guilt, we know that our decision was right . . . for all of us. For a short time he brought joy into our home and will never ever be forgotten.[16]

This is a strange story of mixed emotions and confused moral thinking, but it illustrates as well as anything could the way in which abortion is now candidly seen by many of its advocates as a case of ante-natal euthanasia. The Goodings had a baby, Wreford; and because he had Down's Syndrome they consented to his death. In this artless telling it is clearly irrelevant that his life was taken *in utero*.

This recent shift in the perception of ante-natal life may be attributed to a number of causes, and is more obvious in popular and public controversy than in scholarly discussion. It has been evident in recent public debate in both the United States and the United Kingdom. Fifteen or twenty years ago the liberal abortion lobby was insistent that the fetus was a 'cluster of cells' or a 'lump of jelly'. There could be no question of conceding the human status of the fetus, since so to concede would be to concede the debate. This is not now the favoured language of those who argue for liberal abortion. A number of reasons may be offered. For one thing, it is now much more difficult to sustain such a position, since there is better public information in matters of embryology and fetology – thanks to widespread experience of ultrasonic scanning and the remarkable colour photography of Lennart Nilsen and others. At the same time, the 'viability' criterion has been undermined as a defence of abortion by improvements in neo-natal care and consequent better chances of survival for premature babies.

With realism and growing candour, yet in terms that are also sinister, the argument for liberal abortion is moving from the second to the first premise of the traditional syllogism: from whether unborn life is human life, to whether human life is sacred.

Yet, at the same time, the old idea that some point may be determined in the life-story of the zygote–embryo–fetus before and after which it should be viewed in radically different ways – the principle of some 'critical point' of ensoulment, animation, formation – is being restructured to apply to a point much earlier in pregnancy than in traditional debate about abortion. Instead of viability or quickening, we are now offered the development of the nervous system at perhaps six weeks, or the emergence of the primitive streak at fourteen days. We might be forgiven for seeing in this plethora of points of 'critical' discontinuity an example of the subjective character of hazarding any such criteria of humanness, and of the fundamental continuity of a process which comprises so many lesser discontinuities. But the fact that we are now offered much earlier key developmental points in the pre-natal continuum has undoubtedly hastened the move away from a defence of abortion that depended on some later 'critical' point (apart from those very early abortions that result from the use of the intra-uterine 'contraceptive' device, the post-coital pill, and other early abortifacients).

With the passage of the Abortion Act of 1967, Britain led the nations of the West into an age of liberal abortion. Strictly speaking, abortion remains a criminal act; the effect of the 1967 legislation is to de-criminalise it in particular and exceptional cases. In fact, the Act has brought in *de facto* abortion on demand, and the failure of adequate judicial review of its application by the medical profession has permitted the broadest interpretation of its loosely drafted provisions. The Human Fertilisation and Embryology Act of 1990 now limits abortions under the Act of 1967 to twenty-four weeks, but allows the operation in exceptional cases right up to term. It is unclear how this will affect practice, but on balance it reflects a further liberalising of the law.

In the United States the infamous 1973 Supreme Court judgment of *Roe v. Wade* determined the framework of abortion practice by striking down restrictive state abortion laws and building a right to abortion on the woman's right of 'privacy', initiating one of the most liberal abortion regimes in the world. At the time of writing the Court has begun to back away from the 1973 position, and it may yet strike down *Roe v. Wade* and return abortion law to the individual states.

Among western European countries, abortion is illegal only in Ireland, though until 1990 it was severely restricted in Belgium (where it was only legalised by the King's abdication for a day, since he would not sign the legislation). The Nordic countries are said to be the most liberal, though after twelve weeks or so abortion is more restricted than in Britain; and in a number of countries there is either a 'cooling-off period' before the operation, or compulsory counselling, or both. In Britain there is neither, and both would be regarded by proponents of abortion as unwarrantedly restrictive. The area in which British law is strikingly more liberal than in many jurisdictions lies in the lateness at which the operation remains legal on the same criteria as at the earliest stage of pregnancy. Until 1990, the Infant Life (Preservation) Act of 1929 gave twenty-eight weeks' gestation as the point of *de facto* viability, after which there was a rebuttable presumption that the child was 'capable of being born alive' (a curious phrase, interpreted as referring to viability); and therefore to be protected. Abortions after twenty-four weeks are now rare, though the point of viability is often below that and constantly reducing.

In general terms, viability continues to serve as the practical moral criterion, despite the evident fact that the development of *in vitro* technology threatens to undermine it altogether as the distant prospect of ectogenesis and the artificial placenta come closer. Of course, viability has always been a criterion of medical skills and resources rather than of anything inherent in the fetus. Like every other organism, including you and me, the fetus is viable in a suitably hospitable environment, and non-viable anywhere else. This truism draws attention to the flawed character of viability as a criterion of something inherent in the fetus, and therefore its irrelevance to this discussion.

A feature of the debate about the new reproductive technology is the unwillingness of many of those who wish to make unfettered use of its techniques to address the question of what the embryo *is* – though the radical and candid minority led by Singer and Kuhse have no such inhibitions, with their comparisons of the early embryo with the moral standing of the tadpole and the lettuce leaf. In the United Kingdom the tone of the debate was set by the publication in 1984 of the Warnock Report, which consciously refused to address this issue. The Warnock Committee wrote as follows:

> Although the questions of when life or personhood begin appear to be questions of fact susceptible of straightforward answers, we hold that the answers to such questions in fact are complex amalgams of factual and moral judgments. Instead of trying to answer these questions directly we have therefore gone straight to the question of *how it is right to treat the human embryo*.[17]

The Warnock Committee did not explain how it is possible to decide 'how it is right to treat' something without first considering what that thing is. By contrast, the Church of England Board for Social Responsibility's report, *Personal Origins*, itself a divided and inconclusive discussion, is agreed at least at this point: 'However difficult it may be to decide whether the early embryo is, or is not, a human being, in the most important sense of the term, the question to be resolved is still whether something is or is not the case, and not some other kind of question.'

Personal Origins then proceeds to its judgment on the Warnock approach:

> Some of our contemporaries have hoped to avoid the question of the embryo's status altogether, and have thought it possible to move directly to a purely deliberative question: how are we to *act* towards the early embryo? The implication of this manoeuvre would seem to be that human status is not so much discerned as conferred; that social practice is sufficient of itself to validate the claims of any pretence to humanity. The authors of this report . . . are agreed in finding this solution unsatisfactory.[18]

What did the Warnock Committee conclude? Established in 1982 by Her Majesty's Government to report on the whole area of 'human fertilisation and embryology', its report was published two years later. Essentially it covered four areas: surrogacy, which it recommended should be banned (with a minority dissenting); embryo research, which it recommended should be permitted up to fourteen days (with two separate dissents, one against fertilising with a view to research, one against research even on 'spare' embryos, involving altogether seven of the sixteen members of the Committee); the administration of the IVF system (storage, records, and so on); and the establishment of a Licensing Authority.

The most significant recommendation concerned deleterious research on human embryos, and it produced a major political and public debate culminating in the introduction of a private member's bill into the House of Commons by the Rt Hon. Enoch Powell. It sought to ban all research not in the interest of the embryo concerned. The bill was supported by a huge public petition of over two million signatures, and a large majority in the Commons, but failed because of procedural obstacles placed in its way by a minority.

Her Majesty's Government subsequently indicated that when it introduced legislation on the range of 'Warnock issues' it would permit a free vote on this key question between alternative clauses (essentially Warnock *versus* Powell). Legislation was finally brought forward in the 1989–90 Parliamentary session, enacting most of the Warnock recommendations. The free vote was offered but, by a small majority, deleterious embryo research was approved.

The international significance of the Warnock Report derives partly from the technical lead which was established in Britain, where the first successful human *in vitro* fertilisation was carried out. If promptly enacted, it might have set a more discernible trend in other countries, where a wide variety of responses has been recorded. The compromise enshrined in the Warnock Report is broadly acceptable to the medical–scientific community, whose private view seems to be that it is a first step in the habilitation of the new reproductive technology in an anxious society. Critics have argued that by accepting with limitations everything that the scientists wished to do (surrogacy alone excluded), the Warnock Committee engaged in little else than an exercise in public relations.

One of the most striking alternative responses to the new technology has come from the Parliamentary Assembly of the Council of Europe, which has recommended that we should 'forbid any creation of human embryos by fertilisation in vitro for the purposes of research during their life or after death' (1986). This has been followed by the more significant 1989 report of CAHBI (the Council of Europe's *ad hoc* bioethics committee, responsible to the Council of Ministers) which also recommended, by majority vote, that embryo research should be banned.

In Germany, as we note elsewhere, highly restrictive legislation is in process, though there is uncertainty as to the implications of German re-unification for bioethics legislation (the East German tradition has favoured liberal abortion).

In Norway, a generally restrictive act is in force, prohibiting research on embryos and limiting IVF to use within marriage with the gametes of the couple concerned. In the Republic of Ireland the provisions are similar.

In Denmark and in Spain neither experimentation nor freezing is presently permitted. In Denmark an ethical council has been established to make proposals for legislation over a range of bioethical issues. Its mandate has caused controversy, since it states that it will 'build on the basis that human life takes its beginning at the time of conception'. Its 1989 report recommends highly restrictive legislation.

We have noted that the Warnock Committee consciously decided not to answer the question: *What kind of being is the human embryo?* Given that they did pose this question, their reluctance is curious. At first sight it may appear a question hardly requiring an answer, since it seems to carry its own. It is (of course) a *human* being, at its earliest stage of biological development. From the point of view of the taxonomy of species, it is a member of *Homo sapiens*. The human embryo is therefore the same kind of being that I am and you are. It is – we must go on to say he is, she is, – one of us.

For, has anyone ever before asked the question: *What kind of being is the chimpanzee embryo?* This may be the first time these words have been strung together in a book. And why? No one asks the question because everyone – anyone who may be interested, that is – has an answer before the question is formulated. The chimpanzee embryo is a tiny but total chimpanzee. And if the primitive embryology of an earlier generation had left the matter in any doubt, the embryology and genetics of recent years, crowned by the ocular proof of IVF itself, has dispelled it. What is the product of chimpanzee conception, but a chimpanzee?

Is it possible that in the case of man it is different? When humans come together in the act of sexual reproduction, is *Homo sapiens* alone among mammals in not immediately reproducing *himself*? It is tediously obvious, is it not? It has, however, the virtue of indicating the kind of problem lying behind the seemingly (and actually) simple question of identification. Should we treat the human embryo in accordance with its (his, her) own nature or, if not, what grounds do we have for treating it/him/her otherwise?

That is the fundamental question, and in the light of it much discussion of the nature of the embryo takes on an appearance of deceit. The many criteria of discontinuity which are purported to differentiate the early embryo from the rest of us may be seen as an elaborate smokescreen, laid down unconsciously or otherwise. In no mammalian species is the product of conception a *tertium quid*, a third thing poised between its parental species and every other in a limbo of mere potentiality. The argument is about the kind of treatment that this, our kind of being, should receive at a particular stage in the process of maturation. May it/he/she be held to lie outside the Queensberry Rules of bioethical tradition, and so be a fit subject for human experimentation that is both involuntary and fatally deleterious?

A candid admission of the actual character of the embryo as 'one of us' immediately raises the stakes in the debate, and explains the *force majeure* which led the Warnock Committee to avoid the question altogether. It ceases to be a debate about the identity of this tiny laboratory item which is suddenly available to us, as if it had just been discovered, or indeed invented; and it becomes a harrowing trial of our concept of what it is to be human. The old ethical tradition of the sanctity of life and the dignity of the individual is opened to fundamental revision. Are there human beings whose lives lie outside the pale of sacredness? Are there arguments which will avail to put some human beings there? The debate is not finally about embryos, but about the character of the humane medical tradition and the concept of the dignity and inviolability of human being which lie at its root.

But what of the 'potential' character of the human life of the embryo? Does this qualify its moral standing? No one doubts that the embryo is potentially a fetus, a neo-nate, an infant, an adolescent, a mature adult – and finally a corpse. Some have suggested that the potential of the embryo is reason for denying it high status. Singer and Kuhse, in their vigorous advocacy of a 'low' view of the embryo in the Monash symposium *Test-tube Babies*, go so far as to make the extravagant claim that 'everything that can be said about the potential of the embryo can also be said about the potential of the ovum and the sperm'.[19] Everything? We are plainly dealing in this comparison with unequal and divergent concepts of potentiality, and they are being confused. There is of course a potential in the case of the separate gametes, but it is the potential of each gamete and of the gametes considered together to become something else: something new and different in kind, not a gamete, or two gametes, but a human being. It is a potential better expressed in terms of mere 'possibility'. So Peter Byrne, in his philosophical essay in the symposium *The Status of the Human Embryo*, writes as follows: 'The possibility that an ovum will become a person depends upon external intervention (fertilisation) which at the same time leads to the transformation of its inner nature and biological constitution. It has to become a radically different kind of organism if this possibility is to be realised.'[20]

By contrast, once fertilisation has taken place, the 'potential' is of a progressive realisation of its own self. Professor Thomas F. Torrance, one of the world's leading authorities in the relations of science and religion, has put it like this: 'If . . . we want to think of the human embryo as "potentially person", that must be taken to mean, not that the embryo is in the process of becoming something else, but rather that the embryo continues to become what he or she already is.'[21]

When the Warnock Report was published, as debate focused on whether a fourteen-day embryo should be the subject of damaging experiments, few people realised that there had already been many experiments on live fetuses long after that early point. Fewer still realised that some of them had been conducted by a prominent British gynaecologist who had himself been a member of the committee, and who wrote to *The Times* attacking its critics and speaking of the many benefits which he expected to accrue from embryo research, noting that the Warnock Report had recommended 'some protection for the early embryo by virtue of the material being human'.[22] Yet his own experiments on very much later fetuses were a matter of record, albeit in an obscure journal. If we scour the literature we find a wide range of published reports of experimental work of this kind. Aborted fetuses have been kept alive for use as laboratory guinea pigs.

This shameful phenomenon has implications in a number of directions. For one thing, once the fetus is on the verge of viability (and that is when some of these experiments have been performed) it cannot be claimed that it (he, she) lacks truly personal qualities. And it is also impossible to deny that the fetus feels pain. By this stage we are concerned with one who is undeniably 'human' in the same sense as the newborn is human. Only with such radical criteria as would deny human dignity to the new-born baby can the developing fetus be pushed beyond the margins of the race.[23] Moreover, we discover here the antecedent fulfilment of some of the direst predictions of Warnock's critics. If leading medical authorities have already used live abortuses as experimental subjects, the cosmetic character of drawing the line at fourteen days becomes obvious. And we can hardly be accused of scare-mongering if we ask why unwanted, handicapped newborns should not themselves be set aside for purposes of deleterious experimentation. That is a natural implication of the view that their lives are not worth living (which we come to discuss later in this chapter).

We move here beyond the mere taking of human life into the abuse of a living human. And that is why the medical–scientific community has taken no pride in this record of profoundly unethical experiments. Yet neither has it condemned them, nor acted against those who have initiated and supervised them – and taken credit for their results by publication. Let us review some of the work which has been done here.

The general question of the ethics of research on human beings has been helpfully and recently surveyed by Dr Richard Higginson.[24] In the western medical tradition respect for the sanctity of life and the dignity of the individual have led to a consensus that seriously deleterious research should never be undertaken on human subjects. This position was most recently set out – as we have noted – in documents framed after the end of the Second World War. The Declaration of Helsinki, in reiterating the prohibition of involuntary and deleterious research, was not merely reacting to particularly gross violations of this principle. It was re-asserting the fundamental dignity of the human person over against the view that human beings could ever be used for purposes of deleterious experiment. However great the differences in motivation and understanding, that inevitably links these events with those of the previous chapter.

When the Warnock Report first appeared and debate on the question of embryo research surfaced, the present writer, in common with others, invoked the prospect of fetal experimentation as a hypothetical possibility which might follow from the experimental use of the early embryo. In common with most people, he did not then realise that this was not science fiction, but science fact. Unknown to much informed opinion, the last thirty years and more have witnessed a stream of medical–scientific experiments upon human fetuses – experiments which have ended in the death of the fetus concerned.

No doubt there has been work which has been kept secret, or which has proved unproductive, and therefore never reached published form. But for those who know where to look there has been a series of published reports, in the medical literature, of live human fetuses, obtained after abortions, being kept alive so that experiments can be performed on them; and, subsequently, when their experimental value has ended, dying or being destroyed. We could look at any of a number of published examples.

For instance, in 1963 the *American Journal of Obstetrics and Gynecology* carried a report which began by describing the immersion of live fetal and new-born mice in a chamber of water at different pressures. It then continued without comment:

Human fetuses in a closed chamber. During the first 30 minutes of immersion the temperature of the solution was raised from 15° to 35° C., and the oxygen pressure to 250 pounds per square inch. At intervals of 11 hours the chamber was decompressed gradually by dropping the pressure to one half the previous level every 10 minutes, until it was down at least to 15 pounds per square inch, before opening to see whether any animals had survived. Frequently, the umbilical cord was pulsating or heartbeats were visible; if not, the thorax was opened and the heart was observed directly. When the heart was beating, the fetus was returned to the chamber and the experiment was resumed. The periods of survival of 15 human fetuses varying from 9 to 24 weeks of gestation are indicated in Fig. 2. No fetus was living after a third period of immersion of 11 hours.[25]

Since the prose of this chilling paragraph is not calculated to draw attention to the enormity of the experiment it describes, it is worth a second reading. Fetuses of between nine and twenty-four weeks' gestation were subjected to immersion in a pressurised chamber for up to three periods of eleven hours each. At the end of each period the chamber was opened to see 'whether any animals had survived'. If no heartbeat was evident, 'the thorax was opened and the heart observed directly', to check. When the heart was still beating, the fetus was returned for a further period of eleven hours. After the third such period, they had all died.

Another example is offered by Geoffrey Chamberlain in his article 'An Artificial Placenta' published in the *American Journal of Obstetrics and Gynecology*. After the customary discussion of 'animal work' (in this case, work with rabbits) the writer turns to 'human work', in this case on eight fetuses ranging in weight from 300 to 980 grammes, to which fact he adds the note: 'many of these operations were performed in England where the lower limit of viability is set at twenty-eight weeks'. He details the case of the largest fetus, estimated at twenty-six weeks' gestation. 'A 980 gram male fetus was delivered in his amniotic sac . . . the fetus was established on the circuit; he stayed so for 5 hours, 8 minutes,' after which 'a cannula inadvertently slipped and could not be reintroduced'. Chamberlain continues: 'For the whole 5 hours of life, the fetus did not respire. Irregular gasping movements, twice a minute, occurred in the middle of the experiment but there was no proper respiration . . . The fetus died 21 minutes after leaving the circuit.'[26]

Lest it be thought that work of this kind has been done only in America, we can look also at one of two papers published in the British *Journal of Endocrinology* by M. C. Macnaughton and two separate collaborators (J. R. T. Coutts and Marion Greig) in the late 1960s. The second paper is entitled 'The Metabolism of [4-14C] Cholesterol in the Pre-Viable Human Foetus', and the aim of the research indicated as follows: 'The experiments reported in this paper were carried out to determine whether the mid-term human foetus metabolizes cholesterol to progesterone. Solomon, Bird, Ling, Iwamiya and Young (1967) have published preliminary results which suggest that the mid-term foetus is unable to do so.' Again, the effect of the scientific prose is to render the research normal, indeed typical. Yet its subject is a human being, and – in two cases at least – a human being on or over the verge of viability.[27]

The practical and moral context of experimentation on the human fetus is plainly provided by liberal abortion. So an American scientific paper dating from the landmark year of 1973 (though published in 1974) begins with these words: 'With the advent of progressive liberalization of the abortion laws in the United States, it is clear that a whole new spectrum of research is possible in the normal (and abnormal) human fetus.'[28] It is certainly no accident that the two British papers we have surveyed were published in the late 1960s, at the very time when the law on abortion was being liberalised. That liberalisation both made fetuses more widely available and, more important, marked a change in the public (and medical) perception of the fetus. It was a shift from the Hippocratic view in which a fetus was treated as a child who would in due time be born, to the new perception in which it was a matter for maternal and medical opinion whether the fetus would ultimately be born as a child, or aborted – and, perhaps, put to another use. There can be no doubt that this growing change in social and medical attitudes crystallised in Britain in the law of 1967, enabling doctors and mothers to 'see' and therefore treat the fetus in a new way.

Handicapped Newborns: Fetuses *Ex Utero?*

As we noted in our survey of practice in antiquity and among primitive peoples, the point of contact between the questions which cluster around the end of life (euthanasia, suicide for medical reasons) and those which cluster around its ante-natal stage (abortion, embryo abuse), lies in the treatment of newborn children and, in particular, in the treatment of the handicapped.

In their deliberately provocative book, *Should the Baby Live? The Problem of Handicapped Infants*, Helga Kuhse and Peter Singer argue that 'we think that some infants with severe disabilities should be killed'; and, lest any reader presume that they have in mind a severity of disability that would soon bring about natural death, or a vegetative state, they continue: 'This recommendation may cause particular offence to readers who were themselves born with disabilities, perhaps even the same disabilities we are discussing.' As one of a number of immediate responses they offer this comment:

> Our subsequent discussion refers to disabled *infants*. For reasons given later in this book, decisions whether infants should live or die are very different from life and death decisions in the case of people who can understand, or once were capable of understanding, at least some aspects of what a decision to live or die might mean. To put it even more bluntly: it is one thing to say, before a life has properly begun, that such a life should not be lived; it is quite different to say that, once a life is being lived, we need not do our best to improve it . . .[29]

That is to say, Kuhse and Singer construe infanticide, which they favour, as an extension of abortion, with – as it were – the 'critical point' (animation, quickening . . .) postponed to a point after birth. It is the taking of a life 'before a life has properly begun'. Everything depends on what is meant by 'properly'; and here, as elsewhere in discussions which seek to make fundamental distinctions between some human beings and other human beings, the arguments are plenty but the assumptions both broad (in their ultimately arbitrary concepts of the defining criteria of a real-human-being-who-morally-matters) and alarming (since their scope is never easy to restrict to those classes of human being whom they are designed to disenfranchise).

The most candid element of Kuhse and Singer's book is their attempt to turn the tables on the Hippocratic/Judaeo–Christian tradition by exalting the values of primitive paganism and suggesting that they have been undermined – to our loss. These influential writers cite a string of anthropological illustrations of the kind to which we have already made reference. Yet here we find them cited in commendation of cultures in which infanticide is practised as a matter of course, to illustrate their contention that 'we live in an unusual society. We reject infanticide. We reject it not only for population limitation and sex selection, but even for children born with major handicaps . . . Why do we take a view so different from that of the majority of human societies?' The answer lies in the influence of Christianity, and Kuhse and Singer quote Lecky's *History of European Morals* to show how Christians came to change 'very dramatically'[30] the values of classical antiquity. Lecky's words are memorable, and it is a striking comment on the degree to which writers like Kuhse and Singer desire to break with the humane values of western tradition that these words can be quoted in any other spirit than one of gratitude and admiration.

Lecky writes as follows:

> Considered as immortal beings, destined for the extremes of happiness or of misery, and united to one another by a special community of redemption, the first and most manifest duty of the Christian man was to look upon his fellow men as sacred beings and from this notion grew up the eminently Christian idea of the sanctity of human life . . . it was one of the most important services of Christianity that besides quickening greatly our benevolent affections it definitely and dogmatically asserted the sinfulness of all destruction of human life as a matter of amusement or of simple convenience, and thereby formed a new standard higher than any which then existed in the world . . . This minute and scrupulous care for human life and human virtue in the humblest form, in the slave, the gladiator, the savage, or the infant, was indeed wholly foreign to the genius of Paganism. It was produced by the Christian doctrine of the inestimable value of each immortal soul.[31]

Kuhse and Singer entitle their chapter on the Hippocratic and Judaeo-Christian opposition to infanticide 'A Deviant Tradition'. Their sympathy for the paganism which Christianity drove out of the ancient world has the virtue of candour. Yet they seem to believe that establishing the 'deviant' character of the Judaeo–Christian tradition advances their contrary cause. Christians have never doubted the 'deviance' of their convictions, in this matter as in others; indeed, we have sought in this book to illustrate this fact, not to play it down. It places Christians in much the same position as the Hippocratic physicians are known to have occupied in ancient Greece, that of a deviant minority intent on reform. The triumph of Hippocratism, aided by the spread of Christianity in the ancient world (though not so dependent upon it as Kuhse and Singer maintain), has proved the cradle of the humane medicine of the West. Those who seek to reinstate infanticide to a place of public, ethically accepted practice – whether at parental discretion, as (generally) in the societies which Kuhse and Singer seek to emulate, or more selectively, as they themselves recommend – must face the implications of their general unravelling of these values, which continue to underpin western civilisation. Although these advocates of a new paganism are more candid and self-conscious in their critique of the tradition, they have articulated the hidden convictions of many more. Perhaps the most candid of all their concepts – acknowledged to lie behind their support for infanticide – is Singer's 'speciesism', coined for the traditional belief that all *human* life is sacred. We return shortly to this key focus of the debate.

There is no doubt that the wide acceptance of abortion for fetal handicap has furnished a compelling justification for an analogous approach to the management of seriously handicapped newborns. Light has been shed on current practice by celebrated court cases in different jurisdictions. In the public debate which followed one of these cases in the United Kingdom, a letter from the present writer was published in *The Times*, making just this point. In a fascinating response, the President and Secretary of the British Paediatric Association (Sir Peter Tizard and Dr T. L. Chambers) felt it necessary to reply that, while they agreed with the implication (of his letter) that 'there is no ethical distinction to be drawn between the killing of a foetus and of a new-born baby', the 'very great majority' of their colleagues 'do not countenance the deliberate killing of a deformed new-born who, with ordinary care, would survive'.[32]

The most interesting feature of this letter (aside from the fact that it was thought necessary to write it at all) lies in the care with which it is worded. They speak of 'deliberate killing' (not, we may presume, of killing by omission); of a baby who 'with ordinary care would survive' (what are the boundaries of ordinary and extraordinary care for a 'deformed new-born'?); and while they claim to speak for the 'very great majority of paediatricians' in Britain, they do not indicate that they contemplate taking any action against those who are deliberately excluded from their limited assurance. And, of course, we note their extraordinary admission: that they find there to be 'no ethical distinction to be drawn between the killing of a foetus and that of a new-born baby'. The implication of the letter would seem to be that its writers are uneasy about abortion, but the logic of their admission could as easily go into reverse: that if abortion is ethically acceptable, it is ethically indistinguishable from neo-naticide. Just as the Goodings understood the abortion of their son as – if we may so express it – infanticide *in utero*, the admission of ethical equivalence between abortion and the killing of newborns implies that the newborn is a fetus *ex utero*. It all depends whether the logic of continuity is used to build the bridge backwards or forwards.

And it is not difficult to see the direction in which this argument might next be taken. Abortion is permitted in Britain and the USA (indeed, in most of the world) on general 'social' grounds alongside medical indications such as that of fetal handicap (where serious arguments are brought into play, whether we accept or reject them). The logic of liberal abortion is the logic also of liberal infanticide: the infanticide on demand which, as we have seen, was characteristic of Greek antiquity.

Yet infanticide is not abortion, even if of a newborn. It is generally seen as a variant of euthanasia, since it can in some way be held to lie in the interests of the subject. (It is hard to argue thus for abortion, except in special cases; in most it cannot, unless the very fact that the birth of a child is unanticipated and unwanted can be held to imply that any such child would be incapable of achieving whatever 'quality of life' were held to be essential for a worthwhile existence after birth. But such a broad construction of quality of life, largely dependent on the mother's inclinations early in pregnancy, is hard to maintain.)

In the case of infanticide for fetal handicap, it *is* possible to argue like this, though plainly such 'euthanasia' falls into the 'non-voluntary' category, since the subject cannot express a view and others must make the choice. If that is true, the question of the treatment of handicapped children simply focuses a 'non-voluntary' example of euthanasia. Yet its implications for others in circumstances similar to those of the new-born handicapped are considerable. If a certain degree of handicap (coupled with, perhaps, parental rejection) is a ground for non-voluntary infant euthanasia, then what answer is there to the argument that these conditions must, other things being equal, offer equal grounds for euthanasia in other circumstances too? Which anticipates the theme of the next chapter.

The Speciesist Fallacy

Kuhse and Singer pose this question:

> If we are prepared to give less weight to the killing of a being simply because it is not a member of our own species, despite its having capacities equal or superior to those of a member of our own species, how can we object to racists discriminating against those who are not of their own race, although these others have capacities equal or superior to those of members of that race?[33]

The idea of the sanctity of human life is regarded as *speciesist*: not simply unreasonable or unnecessary, but arbitrary and positively wrong. The 'deviant tradition' of Hippocratism and the Christian faith are seen as having so elevated the idea of human nature as to be in serious error. Kuhse and Singer here go all the way, abandoning altogether the arguments about 'when life begins' and coming down instead in favour of a candid acceptance of the idea that the 'sanctity of life' is simply wrong.

They take as their point of departure the idea that there are two senses in which we may use the word 'human', either to refer to those who are fellow-members of our species, *Homo sapiens*, or to refer to those who possess 'characteristics which are relevant to the moral significance of taking life'. In the first sense, 'the most grossly deformed infants born of human parents still possess the human genetic code. They are obviously not members of any other species. Therefore in the strict biological sense of the term they are human beings.'[34]

Yet are they 'human' in the second sense? Here Kuhse and Singer bring animals into the argument. Why is it considered of much greater significance to kill a human being than to kill an animal? There are, as they put it, 'relevant differences' between the two. One list of such 'relevant differences' is quoted: 'self-awareness, self-control, a sense of the future, a sense of the past, the capacity to relate to others, concern for others, communication, and curiosity. Other writers have emphasized rationality, the use of language, and autonomy . . .' Kuhse and Singer continue: 'Taken as a cluster, these characteristics have undeniable moral significance'.[35]

And what *is* that significance? For these writers, it is the determinant of 'humanity' in the second sense. There are members of *Homo sapiens* without them, and conversely there are members of other species which do possess them:

> If we were simply to compare the characteristics of different individuals, irrespective of species, it is clear that we would have to go much further down the evolutionary scale before we reached a point at which non-human animals had capacities as limited as the most severely retarded humans . . . Pigs, cows, and chickens have a greater capacity to relate to others, better ability to communicate, and far more curiosity, than the most severely retarded humans.[36]

So, 'although it may be possible to claim with strict literal accuracy that a human life exists from conception, it is not possible to claim that a human life exists from conception in the sense of a human being which possesses, even at the most minimal level, the capacities distinctive of most human beings'.[37] 'Strict literal accuracy' determines the actual boundaries of the human race, but it is not enough; or rather, it is too much – it misleads us into including within the compass of those who are morally significant many who are not. A tighter criterion than species membership must be sought. The 'capacities distinctive of most human beings' are the clue (though the writers must plainly mean 'most *mature* human beings' to make their case, since in approaching the question of the very immature their theory depends upon a generalisation from their own sample: the argument is circular).

Here is the crucial point in that argument. The 'moral significance' of these 'capacities' is this: 'Since the boundary of our species does not run in tandem with the possession of the morally significant capacities, the species boundary cannot be used as the basis for important moral distinctions.'[38] The 'crucial mistake' in the Hippocratic/Judaeo–Christian tradition has been exposed.

The subject is large, and it has generated a good deal of discussion in recent years – much of it drawing on earlier philosophical writing. Our contribution must be brief. Kuhse and Singer's argument is slipshod in its movement from a listing of what are plainly typical mature human capacities to the idea that the absence or presence of some or all of these capacities determines whether or not one is 'human' in a morally significant sense. The setting of cows and chickens above retarded human beings is, as Kuhse and Singer allow, offensive to our sense of what is appropriate; but for them to answer that 'the facts cannot be denied and we gain nothing by pretending otherwise' is offensive in itself, for our sense of what is appropriate is well-grounded.

There are several ways in which this approach to human dignity may be countered. How, we may ask, does a list of features which we *typically* observe in (mature) fellow-humans become *determinative* of the 'humanity' that matters? Their presence or absence is certainly significant, but why must we recognise them as 'morally significant' or 'morally relevant' in the sense which these terms are here given? Moreover, is there not 'moral significance' in the fact that those individual human beings who lack some or even all of these characteristics are defective (or immature) representatives of a species which typically (as it matures) *does* have them – and, in some individuals, to a very remarkable degree?

That raises a parallel problem: if it is these characteristics which are of foundational significance in granting moral status to their bearers, ought we not to assign moral status in proportion as individuals possess them – creativity, rationality, self-consciousness? Should not the artist or the philosopher be granted an altogether higher moral status than the uneducated, unimaginative, dullard, who may not be retarded, but in whom the typically human capacities lie largely dormant? We see here the springs of an elitism, a meritocracy, in which the clever and expressive are those who count. But what about moral excellence as a criterion of 'moral significance'? How does the persistently violent criminal compare with the saint? Is the abundant absence of virtue not 'morally relevant' to the worth of an individual and the treatment he or she is due from the community? Is virtue not at least as relevant (or as irrelevant) as the typical features of mature human existence on which Singer and Kuhse choose to hang so much?

Singer has coined the term 'speciesism' so he can set the sanctity of life principle side by side with racism. Yet his argument actually turns on itself. Racism is objectionable precisely because it does what Singer does – it divides up the human race, setting some men and women above others – using arbitrary criteria. The racist's claim is that race or colour is 'morally relevant' in determining how he or she views and treats those of another race or colour from his or her own.

In the sordid yet sophisticated 'race-hygiene' principles of German National Socialism we see something precisely parallel to Singer's anti-speciesism. Had Singer been writing then, the language of 'speciesism' would have been taken up by the Nazis and thrown at their critics. They saw their task as that of ridding their nation of those who lacked what they took to be 'morally relevant' and 'morally significant' characteristics: the physically and mentally handicapped, the chronic and terminal sick; and then those who were judged to be of inferior race, according to the criteria of 'moral relevance' of which they were convinced.

That is to say, racism itself depends upon precisely the same principle as Singer's 'anti-speciesism'. It abstracts certain characteristics (or their absence) in some human beings and determines that these features should be counted as more significant than the fact that their bearers are members of the human race. That is the basis of the assignment of moral worth, so we know how to treat other members of *Homo sapiens*. Whichever criteria are preferred, it is an arbitrary business. The only objective basis for assigning moral status to other human beings lies in recognising who they are. However deficient any particular specimen may be (immature, vicious, mentally or physically defective, diseased), he or she is deficient *as a human being*. And human being is significant not simply because it is 'my kind of being', but because it is that kind of being which typically gives rise to the mediocre or exalted unfolding of those extraordinary capacities which are latent in human being as such.

Let us take an example. By what criteria do we identify a dog, and determine to treat it as a dog? Let us say, by its bark, or its love of walks. These are typical and endearing characteristics of dogs-in-general. But there are dogs which are dumb, dogs which are lame; and if we find a dog which is both we do not set up a new category of dog-but-not-really-dog, a dog whose dogness is ambiguous or debatable. We recognise it as a *deficient* member of the species that (typically) barks and loves walks.

Singer and Kuhse's 'anti-speciesism' is especially questionable when applied to the early embryo, which they have compared (unfavourably) with the tadpole. 'In respect of all characteristics that could be regarded as morally relevant,' they write, it is 'far inferior.'[39] For, as we have already seen, the potential of even the early embryo is there already. The kind of being of which the embryo is an early form is human being. The curiosity of the sleeping adult is 'far inferior' to that of the waking pig; yet to form a judgment of the morally relevant characteristics of the sleeping adult in relation to those of the waking pig on such a basis would be fatuous. There is disanalogy as well as analogy between sleep and the embryonic state, yet the element of disanalogy is commonly distorted by those whose ethics require the abuse of the embryo and the safeguarding of the slumber of the sleeping ethicist. In both cases it is entirely unreasonable to start listing 'morally relevant' details without some account of who this is and what characteristics will appear if this member of *Homo sapiens* is left in that environment in which he or she is most at home; because, in embryo (and the way we use that phrase is itself illuminating) they are present already.

Dismissing the principle of the sanctity of human life as 'speciesist' depends upon two arbitrary assumptions: that it is 'characteristics' of a certain kind, rather than 'nature', which make an individual morally significant, and that it is a particular set of such characteristics (rather than another set) which matters. Yet both these assumptions actually reflect an approach to human dignity and worth which is the same as that of the racist. The racist sets himself in a separate category from those who share his own nature, as fellow-members of the species *Homo sapiens* to which he and they belong. The (only) corrective to racism is the very thing that Kuhse and Singer call 'speciesism', the recognition that human dignity is co-extensive with human nature. Their own 'anti-speciesism' is built on the same elitist assumptions as racism itself, and proves to be remarkably incoherent.

Moreover, what is offered in place of the sanctity of life principle is not a *single* alternative criterion – based on animation or IQ or any other factor which could be claimed to have recognisable, objective validity – but rather an *amalgam* of 'morally relevant factors', perhaps present or absent in some degree. We recognise here the most radical challenge yet devised to Hippocratism and the humane western medical tradition, though its implications are hardly confined to medicine. In place of respect for the sanctity and dignity of each individual human life, we have a respect which varies in proportion to the degree to which certain human capacities (self-consciousness, curiosity, rationality, communication . . .) are realised in a given individual.

We began this chapter by speaking of an ethic of power, in which the physician – either on his own behalf or for others – exercises power over his patients. That idea finds its final justification in Singerism, with its repudiation of anything other than the exercise of human capacities as 'relevant' factors in the determination of human dignity and moral standing. For it is these very factors which give the individual influence over others. It is they which demand status in society. And it is their absence in some degree which leaves the individual powerless and at the mercy of others. To raise them to the level of defining characteristics of human worth is to add to the actual poverty and powerlessness of the weak, the young, the defective, the sick, the elderly. It seeks to justify the exercise of naked power over those who, in the humane society, have been regarded as most deserving of the protection of other individuals, and of the state as representative of the human community.

Of course, Singerism is not yet the conscious choice of more than a small minority, though its influence is increasingly pervasive. It offers a radical alternative at a time when Hippocratism is in retreat. That these views should hold centre stage in current debate shows how far the retreat has progressed. Singerism represents a challenge which, like some before, uses subjective criteria to determine which human beings are to be treated as human beings who have moral significance. It seeks a radical re-drawing of the margins of the human race.

Notes

1   To the chagrin of its pioneer, the late Professor Ian Donald, CBE.
2   James Hastings, ed., *Encyclopaedia of Religion and Ethics*, 13v., T. & T. Clarke, Edinburgh 1908 -; i, p. 3.
3   Ludwig Edelstein, *The Hippocratic Oath*, p. 10.
4   *Ibid.*, pp. 14f.
5   *Encyclopaedia of Religion and Ethics*, xii, p. 30.
6   *Ibid.*, i, p. 5.
7   *Ibid.*, i, p. 3.
8   *Ibid.*, i, pp. 3f.
9   *Ibid.*, i, p. 5.
10   W. H. S. Jones, 'Children', in *ibid.*, iii, p. 540.
11   *Ibid.*
12   *Ibid.*, art. 'Foeticide', vi, p. 54.
13   Michael J. Gorman, *Abortion and the Early Church*, Inter Varsity Press, Downers Grove, Ill., 1982, pp. 14f.
14   Edelstein, *The Hippocratic Oath*, pp. 16f.
15   James Rachels, *The End of Life*, Oxford University Press, Oxford and New York, 1986, p. 2. A wide-ranging re-statement of the traditional view is to be found in Richard Sherlock, *Preserving Life: Public Policy and the Life not Worth Living*, Loyola University Press, Chicago, 1987.
16   Christina Gooding, 'Suddenly it was US', *Family Circle*, August 1989, pp. 88ff.
17   *Report of the Committee of Inquiry into Human Fertilisation and Embryology* (Cmnd. 9314), HMSO, London, 1984, p. 60.
18   *Personal Origins*, Church Information Office Publishing, London, 1985.

19 Helga Kuhse and Peter Singer, in *Test-tube Babies*, ed. William Walters and Peter Singer, Oxford University Press, Melbourne, Oxford and New York, 1984, p. 61.

20 'The Animation Tradition in the Light of Contemporary Philosophy', in G. R. Dunstan and Mary Sellar, edd., *The Status of the Human Embryo*, King Edward's Hospital Fund, London, 1988. Perhaps the best philosophical discussion of the question of the nature of the embryo is to be found in Teresa Iglesias, 'What Kind of Being is the Human Embryo?', *Ethics and Medicine* 2:1, reprinted in *Embryos and Ethics: the Warnock Report in Debate*, edited by the present writer, Rutherford House, Edinburgh, 1987.

21 Thomas F. Torrance, *Test-tube Babies*, Scottish Academic Press, Edinburgh, 1984, p. 11.

22 M. C. Macnaughton in *The Times*, December 1st, 1984.

23 For a comprehensive survey of current medical–scientific understanding of fetal life, see Peter McCullagh, *The Foetus as Transplant Donor*, John Wiley, Chichester and New York, 1987.

24 In 'The Ethics of Experimentation', in *Embryos and Ethics*, edited by the present writer, Rutherford House, Edinburgh, 1987.

25 Robert C. Goodlin, 'Cutaneous Respiration in a Fetal Incubator', *American Journal of Obstetrics and Gynecology*, July 1st, 1963, p. 574.

26 G. Chamberlain, 'An Artificial Placenta', *American Journal of Obstetrics and Gynecology*, March 1st, 1968, p. 624. It should be noted that Chamberlain's work is plainly motivated by a desire to improve the care of premature babies. It is a matter of ends and means.

27 J. R. T. Coutts and M. C. Macnaughton, *Journal of Endocrinology* 44, 1969, pp. 481f. See also Marion Greig and M. C. Macnaughton, 'Radioactive Metabolites in the Liver and Adrenals of the Human Foetus after Administration of [4-^{14}C] Progesterone', *Journal of Endocrinology* 39, 1967, pp. 153–162.

28 J. A. Morris, *et al.*, 'Measurement of Fetoplacental Blood Volume in the Human Previable Fetus', *American Journal of Obstetrics and Gynecology*, April 1st, 1974, p. 927.

    Other articles include the following: A. M. Rudolph *et al.*,

'Studies on the Circulation of the Pre-Viable Human Fetus', *Pediatric Research* 5, 1971, pp. 452ff; G. Bengtsson *et al.*, 'Autoradiographic Studies on Previable Human Foetuses Perfused with Radioactive Steroids', *Acta Endocrinologica* 46, 1964, pp. 544ff; and several from the 1950s including B. Westin, R. Nyberg and G. Enhorning, 'A Technique for Perfusion of the Previable Human Fetus', *Acta Paediatrica* 47, 1958, pp. 339ff.

29 Helga Kuhse and Peter Singer, *Should the Baby Live?*, Oxford University Press, Oxford and New York, 1985, p. v.

30 *Ibid.*, p. 112.

31 *Ibid.*, p. 113. The writers then refer to Hippocratism as an exception, though one representing only a 'small segment of Greek opinion' until the triumph of Christianity, p. 114. Kuhse and Singer's attempt to discredit the early Christian repudiation of infanticide is itself thoroughly discreditable. They curiously suggest that Judaism was more sympathetic to infanticide than was Christianity, and that Christian opposition derived more from the fact that the infants were unbaptised than from their being killed. Yet even these writers have the grace to allow, against this slur, that 'the Christian influence changed Roman attitudes to slaves, gladiators and savages, as well as to infants', p. 116.

32 *The Times*, May 29th and June 1st, 1984.

33 Kuhse and Singer, *Should the Baby Live?*, p. 123. It should be noted – to be fair to Singer – that he developed this concept in the context of his concern for the treatment of animals. His has been a potent contribution to the thinking of 'animal liberation', highly critical of the idea of man's 'dominion' over the sub-human animals as exploitative and fundamentally immoral. 'Speciesism' is essentially human self-justification for the abuse of human power. We might accept that Singer is at least half-right in this respect, though he misunderstands the biblical concept of man's dominion which (biblically) forms one side of his stewardship. Christians find in this concept of stewardship, with its implied accountability, an altogether more fruitful basis for animal welfare. But see Peter Singer, *Animal Liberation: A New Ethics for our Treatment of Animals*, Jonathan Cape, London, 1976.

34 Kuhse and Singer, *Should the Baby Live?*, p. 121.

35 *Ibid.*, pp. 119f.

36   *Ibid.*, p. 122.
37   H. Kuhse and P. Singer, 'The Moral Status of the Embryo', in W. Walters and P. Singer, edd., *Test-tube Babies*, p. 60.
38   Kuhse and Singer, *Should the Baby Live?*, p. 123.
39   Kuhse and Singer in Walters and Singer, edd., *Test-tube Babies*, p. 61.

5

In Place of Healing

SANCTITY AND RESPECT

We have argued that the Hippocratic tradition is essentially a tradition of healing. That is not intended to be mere tautology. It defines and limits the role of medicine and the scope of the physician's task. The moral lines which the Hippocratic Oath draws around medical practice ensure that the physician will have no other role, ruling out both personal exploitation of the patient and any ethic which would countenance the taking of life. The physician is covenanted in a three-way bond: to his patient, his profession, and his God. And that covenant binds him to seek the good of his patient, a good which is defined. Whatever doctor or patient may wish, there is no option for the taking of life.

Before we return to our discussion of the marginalising of whole classes of human beings, we ask a basic question. What in the new medicine has taken the place of healing, the over-arching principle of Hippocratism?

The answer seems simple. Many doctors today understand their vocation to lie in a tension between the sanctity of life and the 'relief of suffering', believing that they cannot adequately relieve suffering if they hold to an unqualified sanctity of life principle. Such a position sometimes rests on a misunderstanding of the relevance of the sanctity of life to terminal care, as if it implied an obligation to prolong the act of dying. Yet the tension runs deeper, right across the broad issues of human life and the goals and limits of medical care.

First, what of this possible misunderstanding? Some believe that the Hippocratic duty to respect the sanctity of life requires the physician to squeeze the last drops of life out of the dying patient. Yet once a patient is in the final stage of irreversible, terminal illness, the physician's duty remains the same: to heal if he or she can, to do no harm if healing is not possible. While that rules out any deliberate step which would hasten death, it also rules out treatment which is not considered 'beneficial' – which is not expected to lead to an improvement in the patient's condition in proportion to any discomfort which it may cause; and other factors. The 'do no harm' motto, early associated with the Hippocratic tradition, highlights the physician's twin duties when his patient is dying: not to hasten the process, and not to delay it if the delay would be disproportionately distressing, while in any case failing to heal. Hippocratic medicine has never insisted on the drawing out of the dying process. Treatment must be beneficial, but killing is – for mercy or any other reason – forbidden. Many clinical problems are interwoven with these statements of principle, and we do not seek to disguise them.

A brief discussion can do no more than set an ethical context for their elucidation. Yet the post-Hippocratic physician considers his obligations to his patient not to be bounded by any ultimate commitment to the sanctity of his patient's life. Medicine no longer predetermines that his patient's 'interests' demand that his life be maintained. Indeed, the physician may believe that he can only properly fulfil his obligations if his discretion is unfettered by such a principle. His 'respect' for his patient will include respect for his patient's life; yet it may also include – for example – an equal respect for his autonomy and right of self-determination, even if it is the autonomy of self-destruction. So he would claim that it is out of 'respect' for his patient that he finds himself unable to be bound by any absolute concept directing his and his patient's choices.

That illustrates the way in which the meanings of 'respect for life' and 'sanctity of life', commonly used in these discussions and often thought interchangeable, are actually distinct. In fact, 'respect for life' is an implication of the sanctity of life; and there is a sense in which respect for the patient (one of the ways of summing up the 'philanthropic' character of Hippocratism) flows out of the concept of sanctity itself. But 'respect' can also be used to mean something rather different, a commitment that could be set *over against* sanctity: it is no accident that we find this term frequently used in the post-war ethical statements which have largely supplanted the Hippocratic Oath – taking the place of direct prohibitions of abortion and suicide–euthanasia, and thereby supplanting the doctrine of the sanctity of life. Despite appearances, and perhaps despite intentions, it builds into the medical tradition the possibility of changing concepts of the value of human life and the possible relations of medicine and killing.

It is clear why the term sanctity has been cold-shouldered. It is an absolute, so it cannot be qualified. There cannot be 'more' or 'less' sanctity as there can be more or less respect. It carries a heavy moral code on its back, representing an immovable obstacle in the path of any idea of medicine which would countenance the taking of life. Respect, by contrast, is a chameleon, adapting its significance to its circumstances.

There is another facet to the idea of sanctity. One reason why it fits so well into the ethical structure of Hippocratism is that at root it is a religious term. Human life is not to be taken, but for reasons outside human life itself. As we have noted, the ethics of sanctity are theistic ethics: there is a vertical dimension which holds them in place. Life is to be protected and respected because it is sacred. Not only does this tell us that we should not take human life, it tells us why.

SUFFERING AND COMPASSION

Once freed from the Hippocratic obligation to confine his role to healing, the physician is fatally compromised. The idea that his freedom to take an open-ended view of his patient's interests can serve those interests better, since he is freed from a narrow obligation to heal and not to harm, is illusory. His freedom in fact exposes him to competing pressures from which the Hippocratic commitment preserved him. The more diverse the range of moral options, the more complex the decisions he faces, the more unpredictable their outcome. The fundamental discontinuity of the new medicine and its Hippocratic roots could not be better illustrated. The life-giving sap of the tradition which continues to sustain all that is best in contemporary medicine is rapidly drying up. The tradition of healing and the sanctity of life is giving place to another, in which a malleable notion of respect does duty for sanctity, and healing itself is displaced by the 'relief of suffering' as the chief goal of the medical enterprise, all in the service of an undefined 'compassion'. While such a goal may be best realised by healing, it may not. Suffering may best be relieved by acting or failing to act so as to bring about the death of the patient. Human life may be 'respected' by being deliberately brought to a close. These are the radically new options being taken up in contemporary medicine.

That is the fluid context in which the twin concepts of compassion and the relief of suffering take on such significance. They lie at the heart of contemporary medical motivation and self-understanding. Part of the bafflement felt by many doctors when confronted with ethical discussion of this kind is explained by their deep practical commitment to these very values. The suggestion that they should be constantly subject to a sanctity-of-life critique in the hierarchy of medical values is regarded as offensive. The question which must be faced is why the Hippocratic Oath – with its fundamentally philanthropic orientation – should make no reference to relieving suffering as among the physician's tasks. The explanation, as we have already suggested, is simple: once admit such a principle alongside healing and it will subtly undermine the Hippocratic commitment never to take human life. Of course the physician is called to relieve suffering, and of course he will/should be motivated by compassion. But unless all of this takes place within an ethical framework that is both clear and firm, his job will become impossible. If this is not so, how is he to assess the value of each individual human life, over against the suffering which the patient experiences? What is to be the significance of 'mental suffering', the anguish of psychiatric disorder or plain melancholy, which can be even harder to bear than pain, handicap, and chronic illness – for the patient, and for the relatives, and for the health care system and the doctor himself? And that raises the most difficult question of all: whose suffering is he to relieve?

That raises two important questions. Firstly, what is compassion? And secondly, setting the last paragraph in sharp focus: though it is suggested that the dilemma is that of 'sanctity of life *versus* relief of suffering', about whose suffering do we speak?

Compassion is a curious word. We tend to consider it a virtue, and it would seem to follow that anything done out of compassion must be good. Yet the dictionary defines compassion not as a virtue but as an emotion, a feeling. Plainly it is a feeling which often leads to virtuous conduct, but it may not. The moral framework of someone overcome with compassion may be evil, or there may be misunderstanding of the situation which has evoked compassion. Examples could be multiplied. Granny comforts the little boy with sweets when she finds him crying. Yet in so doing (knowingly or not) she undermines the authority of his mother, since he is crying precisely because she has refused to give him any. Relief workers in situations of famine have always to balance the need for food aid against the danger of creating a culture of dependence and ensuring long-term disaster. The bank clerk turns to fraud to provide for his widowed mother. The role of compassion in sensitising someone to the experiences of another and producing fellow-*feeling* is, in effect, a short-circuiting of the process of moral reflection. The result will be good or bad in proportion to the understanding and the morality of the one who is compassionate. So, while compassion may suggest a course of action, it does not free us from the need to assess it on the basis of moral principle. Compassion may offer a plea in mitigation, may suggest a truly exceptional case, may lead us to revise our principles; but in itself it fails to offer a moral account of an action under scrutiny. Where it is cast in that role, it can readily mislead.

Secondly, we ask: whose suffering are we seeking to relieve? Those who set up the dilemma in terms of sanctity *versus* relief of suffering imply, and may believe, that the debate is about one and the same person: I am obliged to relieve this person's suffering, and that may qualify the sanctity I accord to his or her life. In some cases this is clearly the position, and – however it is resolved – the dilemma is real and undoubtedly serious. But in many cases it is not so simple. The 'relief of suffering' has become a smokescreen for easy ethical options, in which the physician accedes to pressure and takes the life of one person since that is in the interests of another. There is an exercise of power and a denial of justice in the guise of clinical decision-making.

Abortion offers an obvious example, since most abortions represent clear cases of the taking of one life in the interests of another. Sometimes it could be argued that the child has an interest in not being born – in cases of serious fetal handicap, rape, serious social grounds, and so forth. This is not the place to pursue that argument, though we may point out that here, as in the case of the euthanasia of the elderly and chronic sick (to which we shall shortly turn), the weighing of interests is complex and subtle. It is too easy to be deceived into assigning to the interests of an incompetent, and therefore silent, patient something which in fact lies buried in the undeclared interests of a third party. Even if we grant, for the sake of argument, that there are serious cases in which abortion could be claimed to be in the fetal interest, it would generally remain a secondary factor. And the typical social abortion is unashamedly in the interests of the mother, and others. In order to relieve her putative suffering, the sanctity of the life of her child is forfeit.

In certain cases the maternal suffering is palpable (there may be a serious threat to health), but in many more the use of the word 'suffering' here is as a cipher for inconvenience. It may be major inconvenience (as in the case of the pregnant student), it may be minor (the threat to a planned holiday). The point is this: we have departed from any distinct idea of *suffering*, and we have begun to deal in convenience and inconvenience – the broad language of *interests*. We are setting the interests of the mother against the life of the baby. It could be in her interests, narrowly understood, to be rid of the prospect of giving birth to the child she has conceived. But we have left far behind any balancing of sanctity against suffering; not only has the suffering been transferred, it has ceased to be suffering at all. It is in the interests of another that this life should no more be held sacred. That is a candid description of the moral logic of liberal abortion. Of course, its critics are accused of lacking compassion for women whose pregnancy is perceived as a personal disaster. This may sometimes be true, but it misses the point. Compassion does not carry its own solution. A woman may perceive her interests to lie in the termination of her pregnancy, but we should be under no illusion. Concern to relieve human suffering has given place to a power play in which the mother's interests triumph relentlessly over those of her fetus.

We have suggested that liberal abortion offers an example of the use of the relief of suffering as a counter to the sanctity of life. Of course, those who deny human dignity to the fetus will see this as a mere begging of the question. We turn next to the issue of euthanasia. Here there is no dispute as to the human character of the life that is being taken.

Though euthanasia is a single word it can refer to widely diverse ideas. We turn later to the voluntary/non-voluntary/involuntary distinction. Any individual case can be highly complex, especially where the competing interests of different parties need to be disentangled. Even in a typical case, questions of motivation are hardly straightforward, and there are interests at stake other than those of the patient. Even where there is no conscious motivation other than that of relieving the suffering of the patient, assessments from different perspectives could lead to radically different conclusions. One of the major practical difficulties in the way of legislative provision for euthanasia lies precisely here. Many people can stand to gain when someone dies – financially, emotionally or simply in terms of domestic convenience. The pressures can be subtle and much stronger than those involved realise. They are by no means limited to the narrow area of inheritance. There are several different parties whose suffering a patient's death may relieve.

The relatives are the most obvious candidates. In the case of neo-natal euthanasia, in which a common consideration is the parents' desire to abandon the child, their suffering evidently plays a major part in the decision that the child should die. That suffering – actual and prospective – may be great, and it should not be minimised. Yet it is their suffering, not the suffering of the child. The child too may be suffering, or he or she may not. In the case of Down's Syndrome, as is well known, the child in earlier, as in later, life will cause trouble and inconvenience to others, but is characteristically happy – happier, typically, than a 'normal' child. In other cases, the sheer physical suffering, present and future, may be great. But even here it is hard to argue that a decision that the child should die is a decision taken wholly on the child's behalf and in the child's interests (assuming, of course, that such a calculus is both appropriate and possible). What proportion of perceptibly parental interest is acceptable?

Then there are the interests of the physician himself. Here, more than anywhere, it is desperately difficult to isolate motives, especially in the case of a compassionate doctor whose own feelings absorb some of the emotions of both patient and relatives. There are physicians who consciously set their own interests above those of their patients, but we are not concerned with them here. Even for conscientious physicians, entirely absorbed in the care of their patients, it is peculiarly difficult to isolate their own feelings. That is no criticism, and neither should it be a surprise. It is also no problem, in a Hippocratic medical dispensation, in which participation in the death of the patient, out of whatever motivation, is disallowed. In the post-Hippocratic world it presents an insuperable difficulty. In such cases, where the sympathetic suffering of relatives or of the attending physician is in view, we should cease to speak of suffering at all. As we have pointed out, suffering has become – to a significant degree – a cipher for that altogether more candid term, interests. Neither physicians nor relatives have any right to solve their problems and simplify their circumstances by ending other people's lives. Though sympathetic suffering may be real, when viewed in the light of day we see it detached from its object, the patient, and brought to bear in a life-and-death calculus operating in the interests of other parties.

There is a further dimension. The interests of others may go beyond their distress or the domestic and emotional problems of chronic or terminal illness. In a system of private medical care they may be readily identifiable as financial interests, as relatives see insurance run out and the patient's savings (their inheritance) start to be used up. Where state medical provision is concerned the position is more complex, and the influences more subtle, though the growing recognition that resources available for health care provision will not indefinitely expand has led to an increasing emphasis on cost-benefit analysis of medical spending. The care of the terminal and chronic sick, and especially the elderly, has never had pride of place in health care provision.

It now finds itself under increasing pressure. Where cure is not possible, or where it offers only a return to 'unproductive' old age, these value-for-money approaches to resource allocation have the effect of drawing attention to an area of seemingly fruitless expenditure.

There is nothing inherently wrong with analysing how money is spent on health care, with a view to making more informed choices, especially when those resources are being squeezed by growing demand and a levelling out in supply. Yet problems arise because the exercises are being conducted here and now, in a context of fundamental ethical flux. In a Hippocratic medical culture there would still be hard choices to be made. That is not denied. Hippocratism does not offer its own ready-made solutions to such dilemmas as that between high-cost transplant units and improvements in the quality of institutional care for the handicapped, but a framework within which such problems may be addressed. It does suggest that there should be balance and proportion, out of respect for the dignity of all classes of those in need of medical aid. Yet the decay of the Hippocratic consensus has removed the moral bench-marks and made it possible, for example, to use the interesting notion of the QALY (Quality Adjusted Life Year) as a value-for-money indicator – telling us how many years of what *quality* we may expect for the expenditure of £1 on this or on that.

The problem of scarce resources is one that must be faced even in the wealthiest medical systems – where, as Britain's National Health Service experience has dramatically shown, increased supply leads to even greater increases in demand. When planning decisions must be taken – often at some distance from the clinical situation – cost-benefit analysis fulfils an inevitable role in informing the policy-maker and manager (as well as the ethicist) of the implications of resource management options. To that extent, the QALY model is enlightening, since it purports to offer a framework in which such decisions may be made both efficiently and ethically. The problem lies in the ethics which the theory supposes – that when confronted with a handicapped person and a fit person or with a young person and a middle-aged person, the fit and the young, *ceteris paribus*, have first call on resources – since they offer a better combination of 'life years' with due 'quality adjustment'. This is not at all obvious, since it assumes a judgment of the worth of people and their rights that is dependent upon both 'years' and 'quality'. So it has been argued that in such circumstances of simple choice (for kidney dialysis, for example) either the drawing of lots or a first-come-first-served approach is to be preferred. To say that does not dispose of some very difficult priority problems, but it does suggest that one very plausible way of resolving them is fraught with unacceptable assumptions.

Clearly that discussion spills over into the subject of this chapter. Faced with limited resources, doctors must weigh up priorities in the use of beds, nursing staff and theatre time. The shift from general priority decisions to the conscious assessment of individual cases as worthy of treatment or non-treatment – or treatment to death – is alarming. It suggests that there is a further factor under 'relief of suffering': the interests of those with no direct concern in this case – the interests of 'society'. It is not in the interests of the community that this patient should continue to live. The 'suffering' of society must be 'relieved' by this patient's forfeiture of the resources of medicine; and therefore of life.

So whose is the suffering? The motives may be many, and mixed, and hard to disentangle. The one sure conclusion is that in the clinical situation justice demands that there must be someone to speak for the patient, who is otherwise disenfranchised and at the mercy of the power of the physician, the relatives, the state. Down many centuries there has been one such person, whose fundamental securing of 'patients' rights' shaped the character of modern medicine so signally that, as we have noted Margaret Mead observe, he marked one of the turning-points in the history of western civilisation.[1] His name, of course, is Hippocrates, and it was to cut through this tangle of motivation and interests that he decreed that physicians should play no part in decisions for death.

Hippocratic ethics offered a bulwark against any other medical practice than that which was finally in the patient's interests, for at its heart lay the dignity of human life and ideas of justice and respect. With the new compassion it is otherwise, for at root it is that of veterinary medicine – both in the unqualified place it accords to the principle of relieving suffering, and in its being increasingly prepared to accept the convenience of one person as justification for taking the life of another. In all this, of course, there is 'respect' for life, but that is also the hallmark of veterinary ethics. The problem is that respect is relative – relative, above all, to the character of the patient. By stepping back from the principle of the sanctity of life, the new medicine has assigned to every patient something of the ambiguity of the fetus. Human life is both like and unlike animal life, both the appropriate and the inappropriate subject of medical practice according to the veterinary analogy. The patient, from one perspective, remains a person, but from another he or she has become simply an animal, to be treated with compassion. This permits the doctor to take the patient's life; it may even compel him. The perspectives flip from the one to the other, and it is small wonder that physician and patient can be confused and both alike subject to decisive pressures from outside their own relationship.

THE OPTION OF EUTHANASIA

As we saw in our discussion of the context of Hippocratic medicine in Greek antiquity, euthanasia is nothing new. The Hippocratic Oath explicitly commits the physician to refuse to provide lethal drugs to patients – to refuse to collaborate in the death of the patient, even at the patient's request. Edelstein himself notes that this is the equivalent of 'voluntary euthanasia' (despite its classical appearance, the term euthanasia was not coined in classical times – it would undoubtedly have made an appearance in the text of the Oath had it been in use!)[2]

The Hippocratic prohibition is absolute. It applies even when the patient's own suffering is great and there is nothing else that the physician can do in granting relief. Like the rest of the Oath, this provision is to be understood as targeted at contemporary practices. There were physicians in ancient Greece who thought otherwise, and – when the Hippocratic manifesto was launched – they were apparently in the majority. If that was the Hippocratic perspective on medically assisted suicide, *a fortiori* the physician would take no part in an act of mercy-killing.

The euthanasia debate today is complicated by a range of factors. Our intention is limited: to sketch the outlines of

Hippocratic concern in the face of a variety of euthanasia options, and to suggest the logic of the Hippocratic position. 'Euthanasia' is here understood as either 'passive' or 'active' – that is, mercy-killing by acts of commission or omission where the intention is to bring about or to hasten the death of the patient. As we observed earlier in this chapter, the clinical dimension to the question is complex, while the ethical issue is that of the intent of the physician. If the purpose is to bring about death, the means employed or withheld are secondary.

Alongside voluntary euthanasia, where the patient takes the initiative (whatever the precise role of the physician), there are two other logical categories: 'involuntary' and 'non-voluntary'. The last covers cases in which the patient is held not to be competent and in which a decision is therefore made on his or her behalf. The plainest example is that of an infant, though there are other categories where competence is held to be lacking. In such cases it is argued that a proxy decision is being made for the subject, and that this is different in kind from the imposition of involuntary euthanasia. The non-voluntary possibility suggests that the voluntary and involuntary are not as fundamentally dissimilar as they seem (and as the enthusiasts for voluntary euthanasia insist, and must). For how *do* we make a decision on behalf of one who is judged incompetent to make decisions for him or her self – if, in place of an agreed framework for ethics, we have competing options?

The argument for voluntary euthanasia is an argument from autonomy. It involves the acceptance of elements of an argument for suicide, but maintains it is distinct from an argument that any competent person should be permitted, with the assistance of a physician, to take his or her life. How is it saved from this (indefensible) position? By a qualification: the one who seeks euthanasia and qualifies is someone whose life conforms to some objective criteria of candidature; whose life is 'not worth living'. If a merely subjective criterion is employed, we are faced with an undiscriminating endorsement of suicide. A. J. Dyck has put this well:

> If in principle a person can take his or her own life whenever he or she no longer finds it meaningful, there is nothing in principle that

prevents anyone from taking his or her life, no matter what the circumstances. For if the decision hinges on whether one regards his or her own life as meaningful, anyone can regard his or her own life as meaningless even under circumstances that would appear to be most fortunate and opportune for an abundant life.

He goes on to instance the case which is so common: 'What about those who would commit suicide or request euthanasia in order to cease being a "burden" on those who are providing care for them?'[3]

There must be something which may be identified objectively in the candidate for euthanasia which leads the physician to believe that the expressed desire to die makes sense – in a way in which the like expressed desire of the mere suicide does not. However we understand the idea of 'a life not worth living', in so far as it is objective it differentiates between the simple prospective suicide and someone who may validly claim euthanasia. Yet, by the same token, it offers an objective criterion which may also be applied to others.

This is where the case of euthanasia for the incompetent becomes important – so-called 'non-voluntary' euthanasia – for it assumes that the desire for euthanasia is something other than the irrational response of the suicide. So there are those who find themselves in circumstances in which a request for euthanasia would be reasonable, but by reason of their lack of competence they can make no such request. Therefore, someone else (parent, child, physician, court) must make it for them.

Is it even a small step from such *non*-voluntary to *in*voluntary euthanasia? If the euthanasia decision is reasonable, so that it may be taken on behalf of the incompetent, what of those who *are* competent but express no wish for euthanasia – yet fulfil the conditions under which it would be considered reasonable (so that if they were incompetent it could be made for them)? What, say, of the patient who might be thought to be under unreasonable pressure from her relatives *not* to request euthanasia, perhaps because of *distinctive* religious convictions? Could not a patient who had no wish for euthanasia be judged incompetent partly because such a decision was unreasonable? Once the concept of a life 'not worth living' is accepted, it inexorably dominates every discussion and erases the line between the voluntary and the involuntary. Advocates of voluntary euthanasia try strenuously to deny this connection, since it cuts across their vaunted ground of patient autonomy. Yet, if they are to escape the charge that they simply favour suicide-on-demand, they must fall back on some criterion of reasonableness. Whatever substantive content such a criterion might have, their case is fatally flawed by its existence.

The next problem is to define the character of such a life, since the search for a satisfactory objective conception of a 'life not worth living' has proved fruitless. It is an attempt to provide objective criteria for what is an (irreducibly?) subjective conviction – the desire for self-destruction. The justification of suicide needs no such formula, since the conviction of the suicide transcends reasoned argument. Between the subjective certitude of the suicide and the concept of the reasonable person opting for euthanasia lies an unbridgeable gulf.

Another question must be addressed. It has been suggested that voluntary euthanasia should be regarded as an act of 'assisted suicide'. Is it simply 'self-deliverance', an act of self-assertion which is the final act of informed consent? This characterisation tells only part of the story. In so far as it is truly voluntary, there is an element of suicide present in voluntary euthanasia; the wish of the patient to die is present in them both. Yet euthanasia, however voluntary, is not suicide, it is homicide; it is, by definition, an act of killing carried out by someone other than the patient, whether physician, nurse or relative. Consent remains, in law, no defence to a charge of homicide. Mercy-killing, however voluntary, is the killing of one person by another. Any concept of euthanasia as suicide needs to be overlain with euthanasia as homicide. The former does not detract from the latter, but truly voluntary euthanasia is both suicide and homicide at once. If the homicide element is unusual, so is the suicide, since it is suicide encouraged (implicitly, if no more) by the patient's physician, and that severely limits any extenuation offered to the homicide. It has customarily been argued that self-destruction is fundamentally unreasonable and therefore to be understood as pathological, a denial of human nature and not its expression; so any expressed wish for euthanasia must be discounted. But we need not argue that here, since the complex practical difficulties of the euthanasia situation prove fatal to the proposal to any who have at heart the freely expressed wishes of patients and who can analyse the pressures operating on the formation and free expression of such wishes.

The story has often been rehearsed. Suffice it to point out the difficulty, familiar in every family in which there is an elderly or chronic sick dependent relative, of ascertaining what his or her wishes really are; the near impossibility of convincing elderly relatives, in particular, that they are other than the 'burden' they perceive themselves to be. If elderly relatives are actually seen in such a light, the wish of the younger generation that their elders take up the euthanasia option must surely prove irresistible. Since those who are possible candidates for euthanasia are mostly to be found in such circumstances, it can hardly be claimed that this objection represents no more than a minor practical difficulty. Whatever legal and other hurdles are attached to euthanasia, in legislation or informal practice, their success in withstanding family pressures, real and imagined, may be doubted. What price, then, patient autonomy?

That offers a striking example of what we have termed medicine as power. If the will to euthanasia does not truly lie in a free decision on the part of the patient, then so-called voluntary euthanasia becomes a means whereby the power of those surrounding the patient is exercised to determine the patient's fate, intentionally or otherwise. Indeed, we could go further. Even assuming a free choice for euthanasia, if the legitimacy of an expressed wish to die is to be assessed by some set of criteria ('a life not worth living', to distinguish it from a simple wish to suicide), whose are these criteria? They are, necessarily, not the criteria of the patient, but the criteria of others. They represent yet another element in the euthanasia power-play, for they offer society's judgment on the value of the life of the patient. The wish may be expressed by the patient, but it is judged by others, who determine whether the wish is that of one whose life is 'worth living' or 'not'. Even if it is possible for the wish to be freely formulated and expressed, the power to judge its validity lies elsewhere. Others determine that there are lives 'not worth living', and that this is one of them.

Which returns us to the bridging case of the non-voluntary candidate for euthanasia, whose life is deemed to be 'not worth living' by proxy. Here is a manifest exercise of power over one who, by definition, is in no position to exercise any power at all. And the assumption that power so exercised is exercised in the interest of the patient implies an absolute judgment both that there is life 'not worth living', and that its criteria are so clear that it would be profoundly unreasonable to disagree. Otherwise it could hardly be argued that there could be voluntary euthanasia by proxy. The existence of substantial (even if minority) dissent in the community – not to say the fact of the Hippocratic tradition – is sufficient to undermine the view that it is 'profoundly unreasonable' to disagree. So there can actually be no such thing as non-voluntary euthanasia. It is something else.

There are few candid advocates of involuntary euthanasia. Yet those who favour euthanasia for volunteers have scant defence against the argument that voluntary euthanasia must inevitably tend to move in this direction. The reason does not lie in an arbitrary slippery-slope, but in the logic of the contention that there is such a thing as a life 'not worth living'. Without this concept, voluntary euthanasia is indefensible, since it offers a charter for suicide. With it there is unleased the logic of euthanasia that is involuntary. Involuntary euthanasia represents the absolute exercise of power by one person over another, a pure act of homicide. We have argued that it is impossible to maintain that involuntary, non-voluntary and voluntary euthanasia fall into separate, water-tight moral compartments. The consent that is alleged to make all the difference – personal or proxy – tends toward the illusory, representing the subtle triumph of the power of another over the 'volunteer'. A volunteer for death must give a fully informed free consent, or he or she is merely a victim.

Notes

1   Discussed in the following chapter.

2   According to the *Oxford English Dictionary*, the first occurrence
    of 'euthanasia' is to be found in 1646, though it was not then
    used in the modern sense, but to mean a death which was both
    painless and natural.

3   A. J. Dyck, 'An Alternative to the Ethic of Euthanasia', in R.
    H. Williams, ed., *To Live and to Die*, Springer-Verlag, New
    York, 1973, repr. in *Ethics in Medicine*, p. 533.

6

A Future for Medicine?

PATERNALISM AND PLURALISM

More than one recent writer has drawn attention to the fact that
contemporary discussions of medical ethics are largely taken up
with questions of procedure. Rather than address the substantive
ethical issues which are focused by technical developments and
general ethical flux, physicians and ethicists alike respond by
concentrating on the way in which decisions are made. The
explanation is plain. We live in a society in which agreement
about what it is right to do is increasingly hard to find. It is
easier to agree on the procedures which will allow individuals
to make their own free choices. With the ebbing of the western
ethical consensus it seems as if the only place where we can
agree is in our agreement to as to how we should differ. So
it is no surprise that establishing means through which differences can be expressed has commanded such attention. The
idea of individual autonomy has become more and more important in a society which finds little else in which common
cause can be made. A fresh focus on the concept of 'informed
consent' as the bottom line of patients' rights seems a natural development. Is this not the key to a stable yet pluriform
medical culture?

The only protection for the patient's conscience in a situation of contested ethical values lies in a right to oversee the
ethical options available to the physician. Yet this – like the

pressure for 'lay' involvement in ethical committees and the growing tendency to invoke judicial review of clinical judgments – should be understood as a defensive response to the inevitable uncertainty produced by the absence of an ethical consensus at the heart of medical practice. Of course, in many situations the question is not simple. It is difficult to define the levels of 'freedom' and 'information' required for there to be informed consent. The principle plainly depends on some notion of sufficiency: the patient's decision-making must be sufficiently free and also sufficiently informed; it can be absolutely neither, and there will be serious limits on the material with which the patient can be expected to be familiar in order to make an informed choice. We make this point since it raises a question-mark against the easy notion that there is a simple choice between autonomy for the patient and medical paternalism. For who but the physician can bear responsibility for informing the patient? And what level of information must there be? There are special situations which require special handling – if the patient is incompetent or if giving the patient key information could be harmful.

The more fundamental question relates to the typical case and the fact that it is generally the physician who must himself give the patient whatever opportunity there may be to opt in or out of a treatment regime. The one who diagnoses and prescribes will also be the one who offers the patient the choice, and on whose briefing the patient's decision will crucially depend. But this raises the whole question of the doctor–patient relationship in post-Hippocratic medicine. We have argued that Hippocratism represented a revolutionary re-modelling of that relationship, on lines which placed the interests of the patient at the centre of the medical enterprise. The special difficulty raised by post-Hippocratic pluralism in medical values is that this philanthropic concept of medicine, with its inbuilt assumptions about where the patient's interests lie, is placed in jeopardy. With the retreat from the Hippocratic consensus there arises the potential for deep conflict between rival perceptions of where the patient's good is to be found. It puts the physician in the new situation of having to subordinate his own concept of the best interests of the patient to the patient's own.

We know that the antique culture out of which Hippocratism emerged was not a culture of consensus, least of all in medicine. Not only was Hippocratism born in a pluralist culture, it was from the start controversial, its Oath the manifesto of a small minority intent on radical reform of contemporary medical practice. So it cannot be said that Hippocratic practice depends on a consensus culture, however traumatic the breakdown of that consensus is proving.

This assumption is often made, by critic and defender alike. The minority and reformist character of ancient Hippocratism suggests something different. It first rose to prominence and, finally, to a position of unchallenged supremacy, as a radically controversial alternative to the accepted canons of medical practice in the ancient world. But this is not how we have come to perceive Hippocratic values, since we find ourselves at the end of a long tradition of consensus in our society. It is hardly surprising that our consensus experience has long been projected into pre-Christian Greece as the basis of the Hippocratic myth of late antique medicine.

Yet if Hippocratism does not depend upon consensus within society, or indeed within the medical profession, on what does it depend? At its heart lies a more modest consensus, between doctor and patient. The Hippocratic idea of the doctor–patient relationship carries with it specific values to which they are both alike committed. Irrespective of consensus in society, this community of values between physician and patient is central to the Hippocratic tradition.

The character of these values ensured the rapid spread of Hippocratism in the ancient world, and its unchallenged dominance in the ensuing medical tradition of the West. For these values, while they have been called paternalistic (they are defined by the physician's own distinctive tradition and packaged together with his clinical skills), set the patient's interests above everything else. Its values found wide acceptance. We have seen that they can be summed up as two: sanctity and philanthropy, and they are interlinked. By ruling out life-taking, and defining the task of the physician as that of the healer, the character of the physician's philanthropy is defined in the plainest terms. The Hippocratic

Oath serves as the physician's calling-card: by defining the character of his medicine it also defines him, the professional, whose life and art are devoted to the care of his patients.

This leads us to an important distinction between Hippocratic medicine and 'paternalism' in general. Paternalism typically implies an assertion of authority, a claim (on the doctor's part) to the right to impose his decisions on the patient. Yet that is not Hippocratism. The Hippocratic physician claims no such right, except as he is himself subject to the philanthropic and professional demands of medicine. It is these demands which involve him in accepting a distinct ethical framework as the basis for his practice. This knitting together of technical skill and moral commitment defines Hippocratism and, in turn, the limits of the physician's freedom of action. Hippocratic 'paternalism' is nothing other than that limitation. So it is primarily the *physician* who is not free to take his own decisions. He is bound by Hippocratic philanthropy. The patient remains free to accept or reject his clinical judgment, but just as he may not demand treatment which the physician judges clinically inappropriate, so he may not require ethical conduct which the physician has forsworn. This covenantal welding of patient and physician involves no submission on the part of the patient to any subjective judgment of the physician. Hippocratism represents predictable medicine, medicine that is ethically candid. It is controversial today, and it was controversial when the Hippocratic manifesto first burst upon the ancient medical establishment in the second half of the fourth century BC. But it has always been candid.

In fact, the key to the Hippocratic idea of the relationship between doctor and patient lies in the notion of covenant. There is much current interest in such a model of the relationship yet, as we have seen, its roots lie in the Oath itself. Here the most distinctive feature is its three-dimensional character, which embraces the physician's covenant with his professional colleagues and his covenant with his patient, both alike rooted in his primary covenant with God. The covenantal model of the doctor–patient relationship is especially relevant at a time when pluralism and the assertion of patient autonomy threaten to reduce it to something wholly contractual. Of course there are contractual elements in this, as in every professional relationship, but they have never before threatened to become determinative of the relationship. It is a relationship between two persons, doctor and patient. The contractual analogy always threatens to distort what is fundamentally personal. The elements of remuneration and accountability, if taken as determining rather than subordinate factors, actually make the practice of medicine impossible.

It is in this light that we see the Hippocratic relationship emerging from the shadows of paternalism. A contractual reduction of medical care inevitably brings such a charge in its wake since, if the governing analogy is that of the commercial contract, there can be no place for any values which have not been negotiated. If, by contrast, it is understood that the Hippocratic covenant determines the pattern of the relationship, for doctor as for patient, the physician is no longer seen as paternal. Patient and physician come together into the Hippocratic enterprise.

So Hippocratic medicine can be charged with paternalism in only a special sense. The doctor is not himself making decisions for what he perceives to be the patient's good, on behalf of the patient. He has freely indentured himself into Hippocratic medicine. Yet his patients have also freely invited him into the therapeutic relationship. They are partners together in the Hippocratic covenant.

WHAT OF THE FUTURE?

It may seem provocative to ask the question: *Is there a future for medicine?* At a time when advances in medical technique are announced with dulling frequency, if it is understood as an exercise in technique there can hardly be a doubt that the future of medicine is bright with extraordinary promise. While the high-tech medicine of the West stands in ever greater contrast to the struggles of primitive medical cultures in so much of the world, the continued upward progress of medical technique in contexts where the economy can support it offers the prospect of regular major breakthroughs in treatment. So is medicine's future not assured?

It all depends, of course, on what we mean by medicine. There are two questions, not one. First, is there a future for the Hippocratic tradition? We have sought to define 'medicine' in terms of Hippocratism. For all the medicine we have known is that marriage of technique and value which is the hallmark of the Hippocratic tradition. Moreover, the distinctly professional character of the medicine we know is, as we have seen, a Hippocratic legacy. If by medicine we mean the professional enterprise which holds a high place in society, it is Hippocratism of which we speak. The idea of professional medicine is known only in this single tradition. We have yet to see another medicine than that of Hippocrates.

Does it have a future? Its seamless dress is unravelling, technique is being divorced from values, and clinical skill imparted without regard to moral commitment. The leadership of the profession is increasingly in the hands of a generation which knew not Hippocrates. Yet this is not so of all of the profession, its individual practitioners and its institutions. We have noted the deep-seated conservatism of all human institutions, and the professions above all, a conservatism which has the double effect of both delaying fundamental change and – once it is in progress – of camouflaging its significance. Once such an institution begins to shift its position, a condition of the success of the shift is that it should not be acknowledged – either to the public, or to members or even leaders of the profession itself. It may be left to a later generation to admit to what has happened – and to recognise the new perspective as new. By that time, of course, it will already have taken on the appearance of a tradition.

Yet there will be those who do not shift. Their stand for what has suddenly become a minority position will not be easy. In maintaining what they consider to be the profession's proper values they discover that they are isolated. Those who are most strongly wedded to the tradition discover that the tradition has itself been marginalised, and them with it. Yet the new mainstream of the profession stands in an ambiguous position, since it cannot acknowledge that what is happening represents a shift at all. So not only will the minority experience a growing feeling of isolation, which may ultimately be profound, they will find their sense of identity called into question. And this process will be heightened by their gradual recognition that in their desire to conform they have fallen out of step with the very profession of which they have been loyal and conservative members. The ground has shifted from under them. As a result, they will be treated by their colleagues as disturbers of the professional peace. There is nothing so rigid in its conformities as a profession: it is this which makes it so resistant to change. Yet, when change comes, it outflanks the position of those who were so recently the staunchest defenders of the profession and its values. Once they were conservatives, conserving the professional tradition. They are suddenly cast as dissidents, whose role within the profession must be radical and, in principle, subversive. Whether they can continue to play any significant role within the community of the profession depends crucially on their level of awareness of what is going on. Their insight into their new situation is vital to their survival as an identifiable, if minority, group within the profession, and therefore to the continuance of the paradigm conflict which it represents. Of course, it is for this very reason that the profession itself will seek to undermine their influence, since the profession cannot admit how great a change is taking place. There is no option open to the profession but to re-cast the minority in an unflattering role.

The process is likely to go further. Though it will include some of the profession's leaders of a generation before, the minority may be stigmatised as unprofessional and its maintenance of what it claims to be the 'old values' regarded as incompatible with good standing in the profession today. It is likely to bring the profession into disrepute, since its charge that the profession has broken with essentials of its own tradition is deeply threatening to the status in society of the profession as a whole. The wheel has turned full circle. The defenders of Hippocratism are pushed to the margins of medicine, and regarded as a threat to its best interests.

Little by little, the profession is repudiating its Hippocratic origins, though doing so little conscious of the scope or significance of the (seemingly) piecemeal changes in policy. Of course, there are individuals within the profession, some of them highly placed, who know the meaning of these developments; and who have consistently promoted the new policies. But the candid public discussion of the values of the new medicine – and the open repudiation of Hippocratism – have not lain with the profession, but with those writers (mostly from outside the ranks of medicine itself) whose vision of the new medicine is clear, conscious and unashamed. Many within the profession are altogether unaware of their work, and others regard them as extreme: their proposals for fundamental ethical restructuring are generally discounted. The profession does not see (or admit) that what these prophets of the new medicine seek is already in train. Their vision of a medicine set free from Hippocratic trammels is beginning to be realised. So, though few physicians will counsel the killing of handicapped neonates or Altzheimer's patients, the new ethical writers can see that the seeds of such a policy have already been sown in the ambiguity which, above all, characterises the medical approach to such situations. These writers are unafraid to propose in the place of such ambiguity a consistent and candid alternative to Hippocratic practice. The profession, as they can see, is quietly preparing to shift its ground, though with as little acknowledgment as possible of what is in progress; even to itself.

Of course, in breaking with its Hippocratic roots, the profession is merely following the values of the society which it serves. The relation between society's values and professional values can be complex. The conservative character of a profession will always tend to leave professional values behind those of the rest of society. There will be a time-lag between shifts in the values of society as a whole and the equivalent and ensuing shifts in the values of such institutions as the professions.

It is not that medicine has forced the pace of change. Rather, in its own special sphere, medicine is working through those fundamental shifts in value which have already begun to be widely accepted by society at large. Of course, there are other conservative institutions in society which are equally resistant to change. Societies do not change their perspectives tidily, and this has helped to obscure the significance of what is taking place in medicine. The fact that society has moved on, while medical values have (until recently) remained largely unchanged, is confusing to the observer, who gains the impression that the new general values have left professional values largely untouched. The final significance of the changes in general values, in this case for medicine, is hidden from view. At the same time, key members of the profession, as their own thinking is suffused by society's changed perspectives on a range of questions, are unsurprised to find professional values in flux. It seems a natural progress to bring them into harmony with the assumptions now widely held outside the profession. What is little recognised is that, in the process, professional values are not simply being adjusted but undergoing a revolution.

Indeed, we may discern a two-stage process which first delays, but finally has the effect of facilitating so fundamental a shift in values. First, despite shifts in society at large, the conservative character of the profession safeguards its internal values. Those who rely on the profession from outside are reassured that its values remain constant and seemingly unaffected; and that in turn may actually encourage the processes of change outside. Yet the old values are conserved by the profession for only a limited period. A new generation seeks to adjust the values of the profession to those round about; to catch up with what has been going on outside. The point of this analysis is to draw attention to the fact that at no point does the profession squarely face the issues posed by the move to a new set of values. Its conservative and enclosed character, far from protecting it, has the ironic effect of opening the profession wide to the new values. Only a minority of its members resist, since only a minority are out of step with the majority opinion in society, of which, of course, the members of the profession are made up. Their motivation must be strong. The most straightforward motive is that of religious convictions, which involve adhesion to a special set of values which may be expected to be at variance with those of society round about. Such an awareness of the likelihood of conflict between the values of the individual and those of society is a necessary ingredient in opening the eyes of a minority within the profession to the significance of fundamental change. It is that same awareness which will encourage the development of a self-consciously dissident tradition, even among the most conservative members of the profession.

What is the future of medicine? We pose the question differently now. If the future of Hippocratism is bleak, what future has *post*-Hippocratic medicine, the 'new medicine'? Clearly, in one sense, the future would seem to belong to post-Hippocratism –

to the new identity in which the medicine is being clothed. But is this new medicine a viable, stable enterprise? Will its form be recognisable as that of a professional discipline, however unlike Hippocratism it may prove? Does the new medicine have a future, or will it come apart at the seams as value and technique, joined together by Hippocrates, are inexorably put asunder?

NEW FOR OLD: THE STORY SO FAR

The essence of Ludwig Edelstein's reconstruction of Hippocratic origins is the context he finds for the Oath in the Pythagoreanism of the later fourth century BC. Hippocratic medicine was then, and for some time later, the tradition of a small minority within the wider medical community. This overturned the assumption that Hippocratism was typical of the medical practice of ancient Greece, and casts Hippocratism in a new and vital contemporary role.

Edelstein spoke of the Oath as a 'manifesto'. Yet it was a manifesto for reform, and reform was sorely needed in the medicine of the day. These were controversial values when the Oath first demanded them, and their controversial character has now been dramatically rediscovered.

The fusion of Hippocratic and Judaeo–Christian ethics ensured the final triumph of Hippocratism in the Graeco–Roman world and its establishment as the medical tradition of the West. We have seen in Nazi Germany the one major anti-Hippocratic intrusion into that western medical tradition, when Hippocratic values were disdained by a medical profession which embraced the involuntary euthanasia of the handicapped and thereby prepared the way, in technique as well as ethics, for the programme of 'involuntary euthanasia' which was the Holocaust. And then, with so large a number of human beings wholly at their disposal, without rights in law and with none to speak for them, the German medical–scientific establishment was associated in the human experimental programmes at Auschwitz and elsewhere.

Such anti-Hippocratism was overtly disavowed by the world medical community in the aftermath of war. The fruit of international reaction to the medical trials at Nuremberg was the Declaration of Geneva, which sought to re-state Hippocratism

and re-establish the historic values of the western medical tradition. Yet, in sad reality, the Declaration was something else.
It marked not the re-birth of Hippocratism but the beginnings of
a post-Hippocratic decline. The Hippocratic guise in which this
new, secular and malleable medical philosophy was dressed served
to obscure the profound change which its adoption symbolised. In
reaction to the depradations of the German physicians, the world
medical community did indeed wish to register its horror and
affirm its commitment to the substance of the Hippocratic values.
But it did so in a form considered appropriate to the mid-twentieth
century, denying any transcendent, theistic ground for its ethics
and thereby turning covenant into mere code.

As such, it has proved open to amendment. So it is no surprise
that, in place of the sanctity of life, it speaks of 'utmost respect
for life', in which the relative character of 'respect' is ironically
recognised by its qualification with 'utmost'. The door was now
open for mainstream, and not simply rogue, medicine to leave the
Hippocratic path. In breaking with the three-dimensional character of medical values which is the product of the transcendent
grounding of the ethics of the Oath, post-Hippocratism crucially
abandoned one central tenet of the tradition: its limited but firm
conviction of the dignity of human nature. The Pythagorean and
Judaeo–Christian doctrines had this in common, that human life
mattered because it was given by God. Since we are accountable
to him for our use of human life, our own and others', we may
take neither (whether in feticide, suicide, senicide or some other
homicide). The general supremacy accorded to the interests of the
patient – the idea of Hippocratic philanthropy – stemmed from
this same principle.

The subtle switch from vertical to merely horizontal ethics,
symbolised in the new form in which the Declaration of Geneva
cast the substance of Hippocratic values, marked the definitive distancing of post-war medicine from the transcendent
Hippocratism of the western tradition.

In consequence, the door was formally opened to the development of something quite new: medicine after Hippocrates, the
new in place of the old. These are two fundamentally divergent
understandings of the nature of medicine. In one it is a service,
offering healing or, if that is not possible, palliation to the sick.

In the other, it is a means of serving the interests of the powerful, whether in their own healing, or in their destruction, or in the healing or destruction of others. Plainly, the practical overlap between the two is substantial. That partly accounts for the failure of so many to grasp the significance of the changes in progress. Yet the change has been made, and with the passage of time the logic of the new medicine is set to eclipse the vestiges of the old order of humane Hippocratism.

THE REVOLUTION

A powerful model of intellectual change has been developed by Thomas Kuhn in his influential book *The Structure of Scientific Revolutions*. As the title implies, Kuhn's concern is with revolutions in scientific perspective, epitomised by the Copernican revolution, which led to the overthrow of geocentric cosmology by the new heliocentric alternative. Kuhn regards that revolution as typical of the way in which basic scientific models – what he terms 'paradigms' – come to be revised in the scientific community. Among historians of science Kuhn's thesis has proved both seminal and controversial. In other fields, too, it has been adopted as a means of clarifying the logic of intellectual change.[1]

We can introduce Kuhn's thinking in his own words. Each major turning-point in the history of science required the scientific community to reject a 'time-honoured scientific theory' in favour of another which was fundamentally incompatible with it.[2] How have such changes actually taken place? Kuhn points out that, as a matter of fact, they are the result of controversy – 'competition' is one word which he uses for this controversy – within the relevant scientific community. This controversy 'results in the rejection of one previously accepted theory or in the adoption of another'.[3]

This theoretical framework, within which the revolution in medical values may be understood, is illuminating. One of its most helpful elements is to shed light on the kind of debates which result – and which may be expected to result. 'When paradigms enter, as they must, into a debate about paradigm choice,' Kuhn writes, 'their role is necessarily circular'. Each group uses its own fundamental understanding of things to argue in that 'paradigm's' defence. So they inevitably engage in a kind of circular argument.

> The resulting circularity does not, of course, make the arguments wrong or even ineffectual. The man who premises a paradigm when arguing in its defense can nonetheless provide a clear exhibition of what scientific practice will be like for those who adopt the new view of nature. That exhibition can be immensely persuasive, often compellingly so. Yet, whatever its force, the status of the circular argument is only that of persuasion. It cannot be made logically or even probabilistically compelling for those who refuse to step inside the circle. The premises and values shared by the two parties to a debate over paradigms are not sufficiently extensive for that. As in political revolutions, so in paradigm choice – there is no higher standard than the assent of the relevant community.[4]

Kuhn then asks and answers a key question: 'How, then, are scientists brought to make this transposition? Part of the answer is that they are very often not.'[5] What happens is that a new generation forms a fresh consensus around the new approach which they have first seen as a new and controversial option in the 'revolutionary' intellectual environment in which they have been educated and trained. Of course, there are individuals who, consciously or not, move from the old to the new. They may do so suddenly, though if it is a gradual process they still make a single intellectual switch – it is no sequence of logical steps, since there is no such sequence strung from the old pattern to the new. In a single step, one fundamental perspective is exchanged for another. The illustration of the *Gestalt* switch is striking. It permits of no mediating position, no centre ground. You either see one thing or the other.

This way of understanding intellectual change, however briefly outlined, sheds much light upon the shift in medical values. We take the discussion further, focusing on key elements in Kuhn's analysis that bear upon our proposal of two paradigms of medicine, old and new, locked in a 'paradigm conflict' and giving rise to a 'paradigm shift' which has set the scene for much of contemporary medical practice.

The paradigm of the old tradition lies in its fundamental concept of medicine as an enterprise in which the physician is covenanted to heal in the context of the sanctity of the life of his patient. The Hippocratic Oath enunciates these principles as clearly today as it did when first promulgated as a reforming manifesto among the physicians of Greek antiquity. The new paradigm is one in which the highest value is found in quality-of-life models in which the relief of suffering is paramount. That key concept is widely drawn to serve ultimately as a cover for the interests of all parties who have influence in the clinical situation (patient, physician, relatives, state).

Kuhn writes of the community's 'rejection of one time-honoured scientific theory in favour of another incompatible with it'.[6] He notes that these revolutions have each produced 'a consequent shift in the problems available for scientific scrutiny and in the standards by which the profession determined what should count as an admissible problem or as a legitimate problem-solution'. This is well illustrated in the context of the crisis of Hippocratism by the differing attitudes to the distress caused by unwanted pregnancy and chronic or terminal illness. In the Hippocratic tradition these did not pose 'problems' at all, and were therefore neither soluble nor insoluble in the sense that the problems which they are considered to pose in post-Hippocratism are addressed and resolved. The ban on taking human life focused medical attention exclusively on the cure or palliative care of the patient.

The shift to post-Hippocratism leads to what can be seen as a dramatic transformation of the imagination, of the way in which the world with which medicine is concerned is perceived. Kuhn describes this kind of shift as a 'transformation of the world within which scientific work was done'.[7] As a result, 'the proponents of competing paradigms practice their trades in different worlds'. Kuhn instances classical shifts in perception: 'One contains constrained bodies that fall slowly, the other pendulums that repeat their motion again and again. In one, solutions are compounds, in the other mixtures. One is embedded in a flat, the other in a curved, matrix of space. Practicing in different worlds, the two groups . . . see different things when they look in the same direction.'[8]

So Hippocrates and his interpreters (Pythagorean, Jewish, Islamic, Christian) saw in the fetus an early, developing human life, deserving of respect and protection. In the new medicine the fetus is a mere object, whether part of the mother's body to be disposed of at will, or a laboratory creature, available for deleterious experimental purposes. Again, the newborn Down's child is either a 'life not worth living', a burden to parents, health services, and him or her self; or an individual human subject, deserving of the respect and dignity which is accorded to every patient of the physician. The anencephalic, born to live perhaps for some hours before an inevitable death, is either my brother or sister, to be cherished and respected as any dying member of the human family; or an organ bank, the cornerstone of a transplant programme, awaiting harvesting. And so on.

The perspective of the new medicine (its *Gestalt*, to use a term Kuhn uses) casts human nature in shadow, and reduces its dignity and the inviolability which has been seen as the concomitant of membership of our race to mere arbitrary self-assertion by *Homo sapiens*, a racism among the species. In one of the most potent symbols of the cleavage between these perspectives, Kuhse and Singer can entitle their discussion of the rise of the idea of the sanctity of life in the Christian West 'What Went Wrong?'[9] There is a remarkable appropriateness in Kuhn's comment that they 'see different things when they look from the same point in the same direction' – when they look at the margins of human being; and at human being itself.[10]

And that of course explains the seeming circularity of the paradigm debate. 'When paradigms enter, as they must, into a debate about paradigm choice, their role is necessarily circular. Each group uses its own paradigm to argue in that paradigm's defence.' The Hippocratic defence of the sanctity of life is the defence of the first principle of Hippocratism. Its critics regard this principle as essentially arbitrary. Yet, 'the resulting circularity does not, of course, make the arguments wrong or even ineffectual. The man who premises a paradigm when arguing in its defense can nevertheless provide a clear exhibition of what scientific procedure will be like for those who adopt the new view of nature. That exhibition can be immensely persuasive, often compellingly so.' The defence of Hippocratism has rested partly on arguments that point to the consequences of abandoning its assumption of the dignity and sanctity of the life of every human being by setting it aside in particular cases. Their opponents deny, in effect, that the slope is slippery and claim that the fetus, for example, is different in kind from (other) human beings. Kuhn writes of such an argument that 'whatever its force . . . It cannot be made logically or even probabilistically compelling for those who refuse to step inside the circle. The premises and values shared by the two parties to a debate over paradigms are not sufficiently extensive for that.'

So how is such a debate to be settled? 'As in political revolutions, so in paradigm choice – there is no higher standard than the assent of the relevant community.'[11] That, of course, is simply a statement of the obvious, and is not intended as a comment on the criteria by which communities come to conclusions. But it underlines something which is even more true where human values are at stake, rather than questions which might be considered capable of empirical verification. The Hippocratic covenant is grounded in a theistic context and a transcendent relationship which offers a rationale for its medical values. In post-Hippocratism this dimension is either denied outright, as in writers such as Singer, or bracketed out as irrelevant, as in the Declaration of Geneva and other contemporary codes. The growing permeation of the leadership and institutions of the medical profession by the post-Christian values which are general to contemporary western society has led to the endorsement of those values within the specific contexts in which Hippocratism has for so long been dominant. 'Pre-revolutionary' Hippocratism and the new medicine of the 'post-revolutionary' paradigm are 'incommensurable'; and so it is that an experience which Kuhn has described as a 'conversion' is required to lead an individual from one to the other.

BEFORE HIPPOCRATES: BACK TO THE FUTURE

As we have seen, Edelstein's re-discovery of the Pythagorean origins of the Hippocratic tradition reveals it as a radical, reformist movement. Outraged by the character of the medicine of their day, the first Hippocratics set out to offer an alternative: philan-thropic medicine based on the sanctity of life. We know that those practices outlawed in the Oath were current in Greek antiquity. And while some of them would have been widely recognised as abuses – such as the exploitation of the clinical situation to obtain sexual favours – others were simply normal practice. We know this is true of both abortion and suicide–euthanasia. They are forbidden in the Oath since they were common features of the medicine of antiquity, not abuses but practices widely seen to lie within the range of appropriate clinical options. That was the character of pre-Hippocratic medicine.

It is interesting to note the anthropologist Margaret Mead's characterisation of the transition to Hippocratic medicine, as she takes us back to the paradigm shift which marked the revolution in medical values with which the story began: 'the Hippocratic Oath marked one of the turning points in the history of man'.[12]

She writes: 'For the first time in our tradition there was a complete separation between killing and curing. Throughout the primitive world the doctor and the sorcerer tended to be the same person. He with the power to kill had power to cure, including specifically the undoing of his own killing activities. He who had power to cure would necessarily also be able to kill.' But within Greek Hippocratism 'the distinction was made clear. One profession, the followers of Asclepius, were to be dedicated completely to life under all circumstances, regardless of rank, age, or intellect – the life of a slave, the life of the Emperor, the life of a foreign man, the life of a defective child.'

This telling testimony to the unique historical significance of Hippocratism, from someone with an unparalleled understand-ing of primitive peoples, is highly significant, not least because its author is aware of the implications of what she writes for contemporary concerns. Margaret Mead regards the Hippocratic tradition as 'a priceless possession which we cannot afford to tarnish'; yet 'society always is attempting to make the physician into a killer – to kill the defective child at birth, to leave the sleeping pills beside the bed of the cancer patient'. It is 'the duty of society to protect the physician from such requests.'[13]

So the new is but a recrudescence of the pre-Hippocratic old. The new medicine emerges as a re-statement of those values which the Hippocratic physicians consciously sought to displace with their reforming manifesto. The new medicine is the medicine of a new paganism, seeking once more to turn the physician into someone who can kill as well as cure, who has power over the lives of his patients, to heal and to destroy. 'Society is always attempting to make the physician into a killer,' and in the rise of the new medicine it is succeeding. Killing has been restored to clinical practice and the clock put back to the days before Hippocrates.

THE HIPPOCRATIC CHALLENGE

What is to be done?

The first requirement is for those who seek to maintain the tradition to develop a clear sense of identity and direction, just like the first Hippocratics. From its inception, ancient Hippocratism was marked from inside and out by a sense of being a 'profession within a profession', a dissident self-consciousness. That was why the Oath was sworn. In our day, in the aftermath of consensus Hippocratic medicine, this will not be easy. Yet that is how the first Hippocratics reformed the ancient medical culture. If modern, post-Hippocratic medicine is to be reformed, and the covenantal, philanthropic enterprise to survive and flourish again, that is a prerequisite. These must be the twin goals of Hippocratic medicine today: firstly, to maintain the tradition, to keep Hippocratic medical practice alive at all costs (and they may prove to be high); and secondly to work for the recovery of the Hippocratic medical culture. If this seems a tall order today, it can have seemed no taller in pre-Hippocratic Greece. If the spectacular success of Hippocratism in determining the course of western medicine owed much to the rise of Christianity, we find ourselves today in a world in which the tides of faith both ebb and flow. It is a world which continues to recognise its debt to the Christian tradition. Where the post-Christian society is most strongly emerging, as in much of western Europe, the challenge is that much greater. Where more conservative societies are preserving and defending the faith and its values (whether in the Irish Republic or the conservative religious segments of the USA) the salt of Hippocratism is salty still. In the new and increasingly Christian nations of the Third World there is a ripe opportunity for the Hippocratic rooting of developing medical traditions.

Yet it is important to realise that this is not a narrowly religious question. Of course, as we have noted, those physicians who are most alarmed by the development of the new medicine and the collapse of the Hippocratic frontiers include many Christians, particularly Catholics and evangelicals. They will be at the forefront of the constant controversy which is entailed in the continuing paradigm debate – keeping it open when it is in the interests of the new medicine that it should appear to be ended. Yet there are others who share the concern of Christians. Hippocratism is not Christian medicine, however happily its central tenets have been married with Judaeo–Christian ethical concerns. Its first religious context, of course, was that of the Pythagorean paganism of late Greek antiquity. Christians, Jews and Muslims have readily adopted the religious–ethical structure of Hippocratism and meshed it into their own distinctive understandings of medicine. In an appendix we offer some theological reflection on the character and role of medicine from a specifically Christian theological perspective.

The Hippocratic cause is broad, and that has been part of its genius – as is evidenced by its enormous influence in the Judaeo–Christian West and in mediaeval Arab medicine. At its root, as we have noted, lies a transcendent reference beyond the human medical situation in the theistic grounding of its ethics and the covenant commitment of the physician to his God. The physician is accountable and perceives the value of human life to derive from its Creator. Though that statement is modest, for the Christian, the Jew and the Muslim there is a wealth of theological content with which it may be filled. Yet its appeal is also to those whose religious commitment is less explicit, and to those who have none. That is why Hippocratism could spread through various of the philosophical schools of Greece before ever it was borne to victory in western thought on the shoulders of the Church.

A vital point must not be missed here, for it would be easy for the theistic grounding of Hippocratic values to be taken to imply their irrelevance for those who deny any such religious commitment, though opinion poll evidence continues to suggest that only a small minority deny that they have any faith at all, even in a society as advanced in its secularisation as that of the UK. Deny the theism, it is said, and what need have we of the ethics which sought in theism their justification? Only this: that the secular societies of the West have fallen heir to much of the ethical substance of their theistic tradition. That need not be an argument for theism, but it offers a powerful argument against the dismissal of those humane values which the tradition has bequeathed us.

This is underlined when the implications of some of the 'new ethics' are worked through and contrasted with the concern for the weak, the powerless, the sick, the young and the old which has marked the western tradition at its best and most consistent. As general social values, we shall not readily let go of these marks of the humane society; yet they are the values also of Hippocratism. It is in medical ethics that the dignity and rights of human beings have begun to be systematically threatened. The correlation of changing values in medicine with values which our post-Christian communities are eager to maintain in society at large offers a growing point in our understanding of the implications of the post-Hippocratic medical culture.

The way in which we have sought to address two of the key issues in this debate in earlier chapters offers an example of the kind of argument between conflicting paradigms which is both legitimate and potentially effective. For what does any explanatory hypothesis claim? It claims to offer the best available explanation of the evidence, the best available model for understanding reality in the area under discussion. If – as here – it is offered as a basis for professional practice, it must claim to offer the most coherent and effective understanding of things (specifically, in this case, of people) as they are. Hippocratic ethics have a theistic grounding, yet they claim to be true – true to human nature, the most consistent, coherent explanation of human nature as a basis for medical practice. Alternatives are not simply to be regarded as in error, they are to be subject to the most searching criticism to demonstrate why they fail to be equally consistent, equally coherent, why they fail to do justice to human nature and to medical practice.

That is the context in which we have discussed the question of the nature of the embryo, probing the incoherence of Singer's radical alternative and seeking to show that, even on his own terms, his model of human nature, with its crucial dependence on 'morally relevant characteristics' was untenable; how it was in fact congruent with the very Nazi elitism its author sought to criticise. Again, in our discussion of euthanasia we drew attention to the incoherence of the central notion of voluntaryism which lies at the heart of any credible case for a humane euthanasia policy. In developing these critiques we have not been merely point-scoring, but rather putting post-Hippocratic models up for comparison with the tradition, setting – in Kuhnian terms – paradigm against paradigm, seeking to show the appeal of one perspective by denying that the other offers a coherent alternative understanding of reality. So also, in some other matters such as the coherence of patient autonomy as an alternative to what is widely seen as Hippocratic paternalism.

At no point have we offered an argument from faith (Pythagorean, Christian or other!); though Christians and Pythagoreans will have their own arguments for taking up these same positions. Much has been written about the implications for argument of the kind of sketching of competing hypotheses with which Kuhn's name is especially associated. It is certainly not intended to suggest that the relative circularity which this understanding recognises implies a vicious circularity, since competing accounts are competing accounts of things as they are. It is in their rival attempts to portray and interpret things as they are that competing paradigms do battle for the allegiance of our understanding. Whatever the theistic context of the Pythagorean–Christian medical tradition, it has all along been offered and defended as a way of doing medicine in accord with human nature as it actually is; and in contrast to ways which do not accord with human nature as it actually is, and also (and accordingly) which will not work. For beyond any other human pursuit, medicine is the art of human nature, and any medical model, Pythagorean or Singerian, will be suffused with covert or candid assumptions about who we are and what are the boundaries of the 'we'. How could it be anything other?

The practical implications are clear. Christians and others who share the Hippocratic values are called to follow in the footsteps of the first Hippocratic physicians, and to assume the dissident and reforming role which once was theirs. The wheel has nearly turned full circle. In the West the Christian centuries seem to be drawing to a close. Society is returning, slowly but substantially, to the values of the old paganism,[14] and it is no surprise that the 'new' medicine, in particular, is the reappearance in sophisticated garb of pre-Hippocratic pagan medical values.

In so far as this is a debate within medicine, the aim at every point must be to force those who occupy the emerging mainstream of the medical profession on to the defensive – together with their ethical apologists. They must be asked to justify their post-Hippocratism, to be candid in their overthrow of centuries of human medical tradition, and they must be exposed as they seek by sleight of hand to claim professional and ethical precedent for their revolutionary programme.

Critics of the new medicine must gain a broad perspective on these developments. While it is necessary to concentrate on particular questions which focus the clash of these two medical cultures – abortion and the killing of handicapped newborns for example – it is vital that sight is not lost of the context of these flashpoints in the general development of the new medicine. Above all, we must re-assert the transcendent, covenantal character of Hippocratism as the only ground of humane, philanthropic medical practice. It was its simple attractiveness to doctor and patient alike, arising out of its patent appropriateness to human nature, that took the convictions of a 'small and isolated group'[15] to a position of unrivalled dominance in twenty centuries of western medicine.

Perhaps it will again.

Notes

1   For example, without referring to Kuhn, Alasdair MacIntyre offers a passing application of his thesis to moral argument in *After Virtue*, University of Notre Dame Press, Ind. 1984, p. 8. In his Gifford Lectures, *Three Rival Versions of Moral Enquiry*, University of Notre Dame Press, Ind. 1990, MacIntyre is more

explicit and offers impressive endorsement of such a model of intellectual disagreement. He writes:

> The *de facto* unresolvable character of these conflicts and disagreements supports a conclusion parallel to one already arrived at in respect of other subject matters by some historians and philosophers oi science and by some anthropologists. For just as some . . . have identified in different periods of the history of physics different and incompatible standards governing rational choice between rival theories and indeed different standards concerning what is to be accounted an intelligible theory . . . so it appears that within modern philosophy there occurs the kind of irreconcilable division and interminable disagreement which is to be explained only by incommensurability. So general is the scope and so systematic the character of some at least of these disagreements that it is not too much to speak of rival conceptions of rationality, both theoretical and practical. (*Three Rival Versions of Moral Enquiry*, pp. 12f.)

2   T. S. Kuhn writes in *The Structure of Scientific Revolutions*, University of Chicago Press, 1962, p. 6:

> Each produced a consequent shift in the problems available for scientific scrutiny and in the standards by which the profession determined what should count as an admissible problem or as a legitimate problem-solution. And each transformed the scientific imagination in ways that we shall ultimately need to describe as a transformation of the world within which scientific work was done. Such changes, together with the controversies that almost always accompany them, are the defining characteristics of scientific revolutions.

3   *Ibid.*, p. 8. In between revolutions the science that is practised is termed by Kuhn 'normal science'. The revolution is the exception, and it is the function of 'normal science' to apply the new paradigm, to show how successful it is in solving what were previously problems, and indeed to develop it further.

This may seem 'an attempt to force nature into the preformed and relatively inflexible box that the paradigm supplies'. It is no part of the role of 'normal science' to 'call forth new sorts of phenomena; indeed, those that will not fit the box are often not seen at all'. *Ibid.*, p. 24.

4 *Ibid.*, p. 93. Elsewhere Kuhn clarifies the nature of such disagreement:

> To the extent, as significant as it is incomplete, that two scientific schools disagree about what is a problem and what a solution, they will inevitably talk through each other when debating the relative merits of their respective paradigms. In the partially circular arguments that regularly result, each paradigm will be shown to satisfy more or less the criteria dictated by its opponents. There are other reasons, too, for the incompleteness of logical contact that consistently characterizes paradigm debates. For example, since no paradigm ever solves all the problems it defines and since no two paradigms leave all the same problems unsolved, paradigm debates always involve the question: Which problems is it more significant to have solved? [*Ibid.*, pp. 108ff.]

There is an irreducible degree of circularity in paradigm debates.'Neither side will grant all the non-empirical assumptions that the other needs in order to make its case.' (*Ibid.*, p. 147.) Kuhn continues:

> Collectively these reasons have been described as the incommensurability of pre- and post-revolutionary normal-scientific traditions. In the first place, the proponents of competing paradigms will often disagree about the list of problems that any candidate for paradigm must resolve. Their standards or their definitions of science are not all the same.

Indeed,

> The proponents of competing paradigms practice their trades in different worlds. One contains constrained bodies

that fall slowly, the other pendulums that repeat their motion again and again. In one, solutions are compounds, in another mixtures. One is embedded in a flat, the other in a curved, matrix of space. Practicing in different worlds, the two groups of scientists see different things when they look from the same point in the same direction. Again, that is not to say that they can see anything they please. Both are looking at the world, and what they look at has not changed. But in some areas they see different things, and they see them in different relations one to the other. That is why . . . before they can hope to communicate fully, one group or the other must experience the conversion that we have been calling a paradigm shift. Just because it is a transition between incommensurables, the transition between competing paradigms cannot be made a step at a time, forced by logic and neutral experience. Like the gestalt switch, it must occur all at once (though not necessarily in an instant) or not at all. [*Ibid.*, p. 149.]

5   *Ibid.*, p. 149.
6   *Ibid.*, p. 6.
7   *Ibid.*
8   *Ibid.*, p. 149.
9   Kuhse and Singer, *Should the Baby Live?*, p. 123.
10   Kuhn, p. 149.
11   *Ibid.*, p. 93.
12   Maurice Levine, *Psychiatry and Ethics*, George Braziller, New York, 1972, p. 324.
13   Personal communication, 1961, cited Levine, *Psychiatry and Ethics*, pp. 324f.
14   Generally without the explicit awareness that goes with elements of the amorphous 'new age' movement – itself a fascinating, if in some respects alarming, testimony to the religious character of human societies and, in particular, to the recrudescence of pre-Christian religion in a post-Christian society.
15   Edelstein, *The Hippocratic Oath*, p. 38.

Appendix

Towards a Theology of Medicine

This book is not about 'Christian medicine' or the Christian view of human nature, though these themes have broken surface on many occasions and some readers will no doubt have wished that they had been pursued more adequately. Yet our subject has been broader, and – sometimes with difficulty – we have held our fire on many occasions when a volley could have been loosed from the distinct standpoint of Christian theology.

Yet the Hippocratic tradition originated in pagan antiquity, and its Oath remains a pagan oath. But the Judaeo–Christian infusion into that tradition, and the coincidence of Christian and Hippocratic medical values, suggest that there is a major Christian stake in Hippocratic medicine. So this discussion is of special interest to Christians and others who share a Christian perspective on human values. Though medicine, like much else in western society, has been profoundly influenced by the Christian faith, Christianity and medicine are not indissolubly linked. The old medicine was not necessarily (but contingently) a Christian medicine. As we have pointed out, it first arose in the context of pre-Christian paganism. Though the later spread of the Hippocratic tradition owes much to Judaeo–Christian influence, it does not owe everything. The old medicine was originally pagan, and could be again – though the new pagans are different from the old, not pre- but post-Christians who have rejected Christianity and its values and with it (they generally claim, or at least their spokesmen do) all religion. So the new paganism is naturalistic rather than supernaturalistic, devoid of the transcendent dimension from which pagan Hippocratism drew its moral power. Yet there are 'good' pagans, whose sympathy for the ethical inheritance of Hippocratic–Christian medicine remains undiminished. This book is addressed to them as it is to Christians.

But to say that is not to deny the Christian stake in medicine today, nor the special Christian perspective on healing as the central feature of the old medicine. For healing has risen high on the agenda of contemporary Christian concerns. The intention of this appendix is to throw some biblical–theological light on the two fundamental questions at the heart of the medical enterprise: *What is man?* and, then, *What is healing?*, and thereby to illumine a distinctively Christian perspective on medicine.

WHAT IS MAN?

The question of the nature of human being – as we have seen more than once in the preceding pages – lies at the heart of the contemporary debate about values in medicine. In fact, as we have suggested, there is more than one question: that of the boundaries of the human race (who counts as human?), and that of the conditions according to which those thus designated as human are to be treated (what are the ethical implications of human being?). For the Christian, these two questions are integrated in a way they may not be for others, as we shall see.

The key to the Christian understanding of human nature lies in the idea of the *imago Dei*, the 'image of God'. Mankind – male and female – is made in that image (Genesis 1). It is this which constitutes human being from the divine perspective; and here lies the source of the inestimable dignity of the human creature. Men and women, in their very nature, reflect something of the dignity and worth of God himself. That key idea has been unpacked in different ways. Plainly it offers a framework within which all the natural human characteristics – creativity, rationality, moral responsibility – can be understood; for at their best these all 'image' aspects of the nature of God himself. But just as these do not in any way exhaust the significance of the image, so they may be present or absent at particular points in the life-story of particular human beings. The moral significance of the image, above all, is defaced and disfigured by virtue of the fallen condition of humankind. Only when God himself has restored and fully redeemed his human creatures will the full implications of their high standing and God-reflecting nature be evident. The image of God will then be restored in men and women to its intended fulness.

Two factors are especially relevant here, if we begin to consider the implications of the doctrine of the image for the subject-matter of this book. Firstly, the image is specific to the species: it is not to be found other than in humankind, and neither is humankind to be found without the image. That is, for example, the plain significance of Genesis 1 where the creation of *Homo sapiens* 'in the image of God' lies in the context of a taxonomy of the created order. Human nature as such is constituted by its bearing the image of its Creator. So there can be no such thing as a human being who lacks the image, any more than a non-human who bears it. The image of God is borne by all, however irreligious or immoral they may be; or however deficient, disabled, sick, young or old. It is not reflected exclusively in creative, rational, mature, good and religious human being, though it is not irrelevant that all human life must be understood (as we pointed out in our discussion of Singer and 'speciesism') in the light of the potential of the best and most mature of human beings. Whenever we find *Homo sapiens* we find one who bears the *imago Dei* – and whatever those whom we have characterised as living on the margins of the human race may lack (in maturity or normality or anything else), they share a common species membership with the rest of us, and have their place on the family-tree of *Homo sapiens*. That is true of the zygote, true of the Altzheimer's patient, the potential suicide, the anencephalic. The move to break the link between human species membership and human dignity – not so subtle in some cases and in the case of some writers; entirely covert in others – represents a frontal challenge to this most distinctive of Christian doctrines, the doctrine of our common humanity and of its uncommon dignity.

Secondly, the creation of women and men in the image of God is mysteriously inter-related with the nature of Jesus Christ, since he – God the Son – is also spoken of as the 'image of the invisible God' (Colossians 1:15). That is, the human being of all men and women has a parallel in the human being of God incarnate, Jesus Christ. To put it another way, he could become flesh and blood since the nature of God's human creatures was already one which mirrored his own nature. So in Jesus Christ we have the definitive human being, taken up into the Godhead.

This is a large subject, but its special interest here lies in the New Testament witness to the character of the incarnation. For the human life of Jesus Christ began not at birth but at his miraculous conception; the Son of God took human flesh to himself in the person of a zygote. So any lingering doubt which we might have as to the 'human' character of human being in the very earliest stages of the life-story of *Homo sapiens* is removed.

So human being is constituted by the 'image of God', and that image is to be found wherever humans are found. For the Christian, the patient is someone who bears the divine image, so the priority of the patient's interests and the sanctity of the patient's life (in Hippocratic terms philanthropy, 'do no harm' healing) are plain duties to the patient because duties to God.[1] But what do we mean by healing?

WHAT IS HEALING?

From one perspective the answer is clear. If the narrower 'somatic' (bodily) definition is accepted, healing is the restoration of the body. If a broader model is preferred, moving by analogy from physical health into some wider concept that takes in ideas of mental health and perhaps spiritual health as well, the concept of restoration remains the key.[2] But how are Christians to understand this enterprise *as Christians*? Is it possible to go beyond simply seeing medicine as a way of 'doing good' to those whose need, as it happens, lies in their sickness? To ask a different, though related, question: does such an account of medicine adequately explain the significance of medicine for the Church? Again, does it cast light on the central place of healing in the ministry of Jesus?

Granted the understanding of medicine which we have articulated (medicine as healing), is there available to us a Christian account of healing and thereby of the doctor as healer? Is there a 'theology' of healing?

Of course, that raises the question of the relation between the healing task of the physician and the kind of healing which Christians have tended to call 'divine' or 'supernatural' healing. Part of the problem we face with this special, supernatural healing lies in our tendency to contrast it with 'natural' healing, rather than to seek a broad understanding of bodily restoration which has room for them both, and to seek the significance of all healing in the supernatural character of some. This is true irrespective of the view we take of contemporary claims of Christian (or other) supernatural healing. The exercise of supernatural gifts of healing in New Testament times – supremely, by our Lord himself – is not in dispute. If, however, we believe that supernatural healing has an important part to play in the life and ministry of the Church today, the question of its relations with natural, medical healing is acute. We will be able to understand unusual and remarkable healing better once we have some grasp of the significance of the usual and unremarkable. By the same token, much of the significance which has been thought to attach to supernatural healing may actually be predicated also of the healing task of the doctor.

From a medical perspective, the matter is debated although relatively clear. Healing is about the restoration of 'health', whether defined somatically or more broadly. It can be taken to include the psychological and aspects of the social well-being of man. For the Christian, spiritual 'health' may not be simply a metaphor – man is only truly 'well' when all is well. Yet the metaphorical element here is certainly strong, and the model employed is that of bodily function and dysfunction. However much we share a Christian concern for the ultimate well-being of our fellows, the calling of medicine is historically and professionally an abstraction of the physical and, more recently, the psychological from the full character of man as he was made by God.

The idea of healing is essentially restorative, so it is dependent upon there being something wrong – something needing to be restored. Healing is a response to sickness. Healing is a function of the disordered state of fallen human existence. From a theological perspective it may be seen as part of God's gracious response to the fall of man and the curse. Restoration to health is not always possible, and therefore there is more to medicine than healing defined as restoration. Moreover, medicine may be the context for prevention rather than cure. Yet the preventative, and especially the palliative, responsibilities of the profession should be understood as consequential upon the physician's call to be a healer. It is in the call and commitment to heal that we discover the essence of medicine. Healing itself is a function of the physician's respect for the patient; so if healing fails or has no place, there will be palliative care instead. The Hippocratic physician never lays aside the mantle of the healer, even though his hopes and best intentions are finally frustrated in chronic sickness and death.

What of so-called 'divine healing'? The term is unfortunate, since by drawing attention to the divine cause of healing in a particular case, it implies that the cause of other healing is other than divine, setting one way of God's working over against another. The word 'miracle' raises broader questions, but 'miraculous healing' is a healthier term for special acts of healing such as we find in the ministry of Jesus. Though claims that miraculous healing is to be found in the contemporary Church raise important questions, they do not affect this discussion.[3] The theological significance of healing does not attach to the mode employed, but to the result achieved. More fundamental is the question why some people are healed and others not. From this perspective, the mode is plainly secondary and in any event may be unclear. Moreover, we must extend the scope of 'healing' even beyond that of miracle and medical skill, since natural remission and cure are also possible. All, from this perspective, are one: the restoration of bodily health in the face of sickness.

The significance of healing is to be set in a double theological context.

Firstly, the context provided by our understanding of *the providence of God*. Discussion of sickness and healing has suffered much from our failure to recognise their place in the general providential circumstances of the Christian life. Sickness has been isolated from other experiences attendant upon fallen human existence, as if its cause – and therefore its potential remedy – were distinct from theirs. Of course, there are some distinctive issues involved in sickness, since it is so closely connected with the curse of mortality out of which it arises, though such misfortunes as accidental injury and malnutrition are closely related phenomena. Yet, finally, every experience of good or ill in human life arises from that same curse – or from the providential goodness of God in mitigating its effects. Mortal, certainly, we remain. Sickness, poverty, unfulfilled ambition, disability, marital failure – every sad and sorrowful human circumstance arises out of a single fundamental cause. So the preachers of health and wealth with their 'prosperity gospel' are right to make these connections. There are distinctions which must also be maintained: health is the normal state of the human body, while wealth is a relative and incidental feature of human experience. They are united in this: whatever guarantee, or lack of guarantee, the Christian has for the one will surely hold also for the other. Where the prosperity preachers are wrong is in their idea that the Christian has any guarantee at all, since he has none.

Sickness and health find their place in Christian experience, alongside other providential circumstances in God's fallen world. And that is nowhere better illustrated than in the story of Job. In chapter 1 he loses his wealth, in chapter 2 his health, and as the familiar story unfolds we find him sick, bereaved and impoverished, all as part of his one experience of providential management in the hands of a wise and good God, but (and this is crucial to the message of the book) also an inscrutable God, whose providence is beneficent but may appear inexplicable. Among the most significant but least-noticed elements in the book's theodicy is the fact that Job evidently did not know of the events recorded in the first two chapters of the book which bears his name – not when they happened, nor when God finally 'answered' Job, nor, so far as we are aware, until his dying day.

The book of Job stands as a bulwark against the naive reading of Holy Scripture that would lead us in the direction of the health-and-wealth package, especially since attempts to canvas biblical support for that package invariably find their focus in the Old Testament. Job's comforters, as we call them, are types of the kindly, religious people in every day, whose good intentions are frustrated by limited theological horizons and a refusal to believe that there is anything beyond them. They apply their naive theories of history and providence to the seemingly pathetic, failed life of Job, in fact a figure of incomparable stature. And they are shown by God to have been profoundly wrong. He himself offers Job as his test case of faith and fidelity.

This is not the place for an extended discussion of the meaning of the book of Job, though it plays a key role in suggesting a biblical understanding of providence and misfortune. Its neglect within the Church is a serious impoverishment of its theology and spirituality, in an age preoccupied with tragedy on the one hand and special blessing on the other. It is hard to imagine a closer parallel than that between Job's 'comforters' and contemporary purveyors of the notion that bodily well-being and comfort in the Christian life are directly proportional to virtue. By contrast, in God's revelation of what is going on behind the scenes, we have an altogether different explanation of the sufferings of this man. They prove to the powers of darkness that faith is independent of just such comfortable circumstances. Job's selection to play this harrowing role arises not from lack of virtue on his part but precisely from its presence. 'Have you considered my servant Job?' says God, when he seeks an example of disinterested faith (Job 1:8). And to Job God offers himself as the sole guarantee of his ultimate providential beneficence. He must be taken on trust.

What emerges is this: the only thorough-going alternative to health-and-wealth theology is the theology and theodicy offered by the book of Job, a theology of providence in place of a theology of prosperity. Christians are not immune to the 'slings and arrows of outrageous fortune': they get sick, their loved ones die, their houses burn down, their cars are stolen, they lose their jobs. Of course, they may contribute culpably to each of these circumstances. But in the absence of prophecy or other supernatural revelation no special significance need attach to them. So we do well to still the conceit that led Job's friends to jump to conclusions about why his life was falling apart.

> Blind unbelief is sure to err,
> And scan his work in vain;
> God is his own interpreter,
> And he will make it plain.

And from that perspective illness and misfortune are alike providential mysteries to leave in the hands of the God in whom we trust. The Christian with cancer is to be understood by analogy with other Christians in distressing circumstances. Relief may be natural or supernatural, it may be the answer to prayer or it may not. We *believe* that for the Christian all things work together for good; but that is an article of faith, it is not a divine safe-conduct through the vicissitudes of fallen human affairs. There are martyrs of the gospel, Christian children who die, fine men and women taken from us in the flower of promise. 'The Lord gave and the Lord has taken away,' said Job of all people; 'blessed be the name of the Lord.'

Which takes us to an argument that is often aired at this point in defence of a view of healing distinct from the broader expectation of a naively benign providence. One recent writer has put it like this: 'Supporters of divine healing . . . believe that physical healing, like salvation, is an inheritance of every believer through the atoning death of Christ . . . this view concludes that Christ has borne man's bodily as well as spiritual sufferings on the cross. Thus one receives physical healing by faith just as he receives his salvation.'[4]

The problem with this way of arguing, apart from its weak basis in Scripture, is that it proves too much. It is not an argument for healing, it is actually an argument for immortality – the avoidance of death. Yet no New Testament writer claims this, and mortality is not simply the fact that we die, it is that we are all the time subject to death and the shadow which it casts over human life. The effects of the cross are as cosmic as those of the fall; yet the 'whole creation' is still 'groaning and travailing' as it waits with 'eager longing'. And for what does it wait? For the 'adoption as sons, the redemption of our bodies' (Romans 8:23). And Paul continues in the next two verses: 'For in this hope we were saved. Now hope that is seen is not hope. For who hopes for what he sees? But if we hope for what we do not see, we wait for it with patience.'

This text furnishes us with a key to the biblical concept of sickness and healing. The redemption of the body is promised, but not yet. We must wait for it with patience, for it will not come until the final consummation. Until then we must groan and travail with the rest of creation. The key to our understanding of the Christian life is its eschatological orientation, an extended hoping for what we do not yet see.

That leads us on naturally to our second context for healing, and that is *eschatology* itself. The final redemption of the body must wait until the Last Things, so what is the place of healing in this life?

The short answer is that its place can only ever be ambiguous, since healing – all healing, however it comes about – is a blessing of the world to come. Such blessings can only ever be partially realised in the here and now. And that leads to an ironic observation on the character of some contemporary debate. If the redemption of the body awaits the last day, the notion that physical health and healing are somehow guaranteed to the believer implies a strangely this-worldly understanding of salvation. It is the custom of evangelicals to criticise those who are over-ready to interpret the gospel in terms of social and political reform, since they fail to do justice to the eschatological character of the faith. The fulness of the kingdom awaits us in the world to come, and is simply unrealisable in the world of today – however important our Christian responsibility to be 'salt and light' in our own time and place.

A this-worldly idea of the redemption of the body itself fails to do justice to the eschatological character of the New Testament. Supernatural healing in Scripture is always a sampling process of glory and the hereafter. The balance is carefully maintained, and we must struggle to make it our own.

Yes: we believe that glory breaks through into this world, keeps breaking in, to shake us in our complacency, to stir up our hope of another world. But it does not break in in order to create in this world an island of the other. In the words of the hymn:

> The hill of Zion yields
> A thousand sacred sweets,
> Before we reach those heavenly fields
> And walk the sacred streets.

But we are still (as the chorus says) 'marching to Zion'. We are not yet there. Though not 'of this world' we are in it, and in it we stay, until the other dawns.

Miraculous healing is presented to us in Scripture as a breaking-in to this world of the powers of the world to come. But a similar character attaches to all healing. For if the final context of all sickness is the curse, the final context of all healing must be the resurrection of the body. And if healing itself is an anticipation of the resurrection, a rolling back of the frontiers of the fall, whether medical or supernatural in nature, it partakes of an eschatological character.

Whenever medicine is being true to itself, its calling is to staunch the wound of the curse, to stay the hand of the destroyer, to secure for life all that can be grasped out of the clutches of death. That is why it is so alarming to hear physicians and ethicists speak of 'letting Nature take its course', for the whole rationale of the medical enterprise is a grand design to stop 'Nature' in her tracks. Of course, there *is* no 'Nature'; it is a misleading shorthand for yielding to the natural process, in this case allowing death to do its work unhindered. And while we rightly maintain that once the dying process is irreversible there may be limits to what the physician must do, his very calling as a physician is to stand in the breach and to deny death access. There is no Nature, but there is Death. The dissolution of the corporeal existence of man, to which all sickness tends and which comes to completion in every act of human dying, is the outworking of the savage principle of Death let loose in the world by the mysterious, providential judgment of God in answer to the sin of Adam. It is an enemy, the last enemy, and in this world it is the peculiar calling of the physician to fight it, and to maintain these frail, mortal creatures to the last, in recognition of the one whose image they bear.

Now if the redemption of the body is the final consequence of the defeat of the last enemy, the task of healing is an eschatological responsibility, a partial realisation in the here and now of something that will finally be accomplished there and then. That is why, in the good providence of God, the pagan Hippocratic tradition could be put on by the Church like a glove. It is why in his own ministry Jesus was known as a healer. It is why, in taking on the healer's mantle, the physician wears the garment which will finally be worn in glory by none other than God himself.

Then the eyes of the blind shall be opened,
  and the ears of the deaf unstopped;
then shall the lame man leap like a hart,
  and the tongue of the dumb sing for joy. (Isaiah 35:5–6)

Notes

1   Most Christians do not deny that in certain and specific cases the 'sanctity' of life does not prevent, e.g., just warfare or, perhaps, the capital sentence. These are cases for which Scripture makes specific provision. Their significance is not to undermine but to set in even sharper focus the sanctity of life. The principle is that only God may rightly take human life. On these specific occasions, it is at his explicit command that life is taken – whether supernaturally (as sometimes in Scripture) or by obedience to his revealed will. God alone may take human life: on these occasions it is he who does.

2   Christians tend to be attracted by broader concepts than the somatic in reaction against the materialist reduction of human life. This is partly a debate about definitions, and many would accept that non-somatic ideas of health are essentially analogical, and therefore actually *depend* on a strict somatic definition of health as bodily health, even as they extend the idea of health as well-being into every sphere of life.

    A recent example of Christian enthusiasm for the broad definition, without apparent awareness of its analogical character, is to be found in a statement issued by members of various Christian bodies in Britain in 1989 (including the Churches' Council on Health and Healing, and the Christian Medical Fellowship). The statement defined health as 'the strength to be human', linking it with ' "wholeness" . . . part of the Biblical concept of *Shalom*', involving 'wholeness, well-being, vigour, and vitality in all dimensions of human life.'

3   The best recent summary of claims of miraculous healing is that of R. F. R. Gardner, *Healing Miracles*, Darton, Longman and Todd, London, 1986.

4   P. G. Chappell, 'Heal, Healing' in *Evangelical Dictionary of Theology*, Baker Book House, Grand Rapids, 1984.

Select Bibliography

The manuscript of this book was completed before the appearance of Owsei Temkin's *Hippocrates in a World of Pagans and Christians* (Johns Hopkins University Press, Baltimore, 1991), a learned fascinating study of the triumph of Hippocratic medicine. But Temkin's concerns are largely distinct from our own, in his concentration on medicine rather than medical ethics. Danielle Gourévitch's very substantial French work, *Le Triangle Hippocratique dans le Monde Greco-Romain* (Ecole Français de Rome, Rome, 1984), shows more concern for Hippocratic values. Both these books open scholarly windows on the world of classical medicine under the Hippocratic impress.

There are two standard English-language works on the Oath. W. H. S. Jones' short essay *The Doctor's Oath* (Cambridge University Press, 1924) is a useful review of textual questions as well as a commentary on the Oath. Ludwig Edelstein's influential monograph, *The Hippocratic Oath* (John Hopkins University Press, Baltimore, 1943), offers the historical reconstruction of early Hippocratism which – for the sake of argument – we have assumed in our discussion. Among other works, Manfred Ullmann's *Islamic Medicine* (Edinburgh University Press, 1978) summarises this related tradition.

In a series of sensitive volumes of essays Stanley Hauerwas has discussed issues of human value in the context of contemporary developments in medicine: *Suffering Presence* has a special focus on the question of the handicapped (University of Notre Dame Press, Indiana, 1986; T. & T. Clark, Edinburgh, 1988).

The most helpful brief introduction to the horrors of Nazi medicine is Leo Alexander's 1949 essay on 'Medical Science under Dictatorship', recently reprinted in *Death without Dignity:*

Euthanasia in Perspective, edited by the present writer (Rutherford House Books, Edinburgh, 1990). Two scholarly volumes recently published are: Robert Proctor, *Racial Hygiene: Medicine under the Nazis* (Harvard University Press, Cambridge, Mass., and London, 1988) and Benno Müller-Hill, *Murderous Science* (Oxford University Press, 1988). A wave of renewed academic interest in this story continues to produce new research, and has also resulted in medical and other interest in the lessons to be learned.

In *The End of Life* (Oxford University Press, 1986) James Rachels offers one of the many increasingly candid cases for euthanasia and the abandonment of the sanctity-of-life principle which have been appearing. Richard Sherlock's *Preserving Life: Public Policy and the Life not Worth Living* (Loyola University Press, Chicago, 1987) takes a very different approach and explores it in the perspective of public policy. A series of books co-authored or co-edited by Peter Singer and Helga Kuhse argue the case for the 'new medicine' with some cogency and a superficial attraction; for example, *Should the Baby Live?* (Oxford University Press, 1985). Two helpful essays by Teresa Iglesias on the nature of the embryo are contained in the present writer's *Embryos and Ethics* (Rutherford House, Edinburgh, 1987), and other articles on a range of topics appear in *Ethics and Medicine* (published three times a year by the Paternoster Press of Exeter, England).

Index